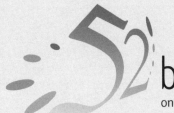

52 brilliant ideas

one good idea can change your life...

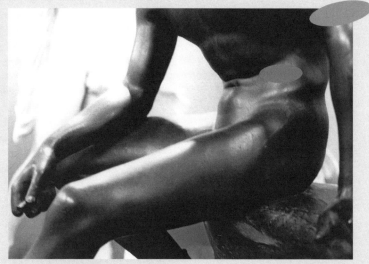

Power-up Pilates

Power and poise for daily life

Steve Shipside

CAREFUL NOW...

Before beginning any exercise programme, it is advisable to obtain the approval and recommendations of your doctor. While you are following any exercise programme, it is advisable to visit your doctor for periodic monitoring.

Mention of specific companies in this book does not necessarily imply endorsement by the publisher, nor does it imply that those companies endorse the book.

Know your limits and don't take risks beyond your level of experience or ability. It's your body, and it's up to you to take responsibility for your own safety and progress. Fix your own goals and focus on your own workout – not what other people are doing. Attempting to compete without knowing what you're doing is the fast track to coming a cropper. There's no point getting the fitness bug only to crock yourself and end up spectating sulkily from the sidelines.

Any form of exercise activity poses potential health risks. Inactivity, on the other hand, makes health risks a certainty.

First published in 2004 by
The Infinite Ideas Company Limited
Belsyre Court
57 Woodstock Road
Oxford
OX2 6HJ
United Kingdom
www.infideas.com

CIP catalogue records for this book are available from the British Library and the US Library of Congress.

ISBN 1-904902-04-9

Brand and product names are trademarks or registered trademarks of their respective owners.

Line illustrations by Andy White
Designed and typeset by Baseline Arts Ltd, Oxford
Printed and bound by TJ International, Cornwall

Brilliant ideas

Brilliant features

Each chapter of this book is designed to provide you with an inspirational idea that you can read quickly and put into practice straight away.

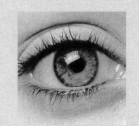

Throughout you'll find four features that will help you to get right to the heart of the idea:

- *Try another idea* If this idea looks like a life-changer then there's no time to lose. *Try another idea* will point you straight to a related tip to expand and enhance the first.

- *Here's an idea for you* Give it a go – right here, right now – and get an idea of how well you're doing so far.

- *Defining ideas* Words of wisdom from masters and mistresses of the art, plus some interesting hangers-on.

- *How did it go?* If at first you do succeed try to hide your amazement. If, on the other hand, you don't this is where you'll find a Q and A that highlights common problems and how to get over them.

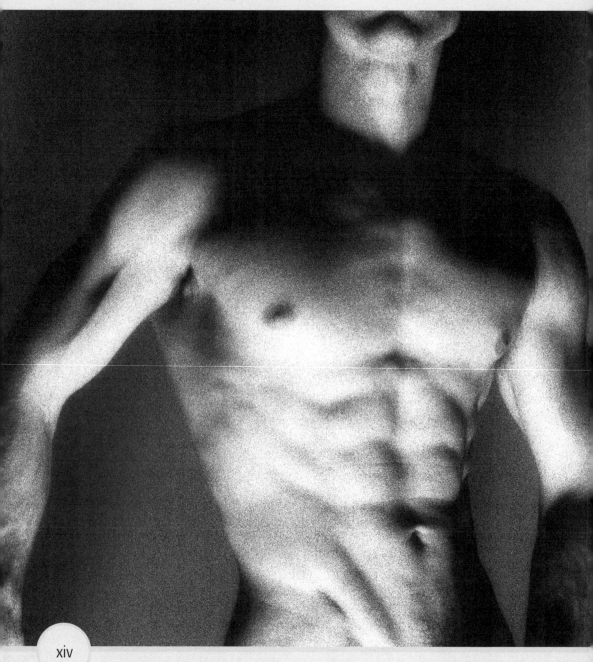

Introduction

Described as 'yoga with movements', Pilates is often now associated with a lithe, leotard-clad clique and not a little New Age spiritualism. Which makes it all the more interesting when you see the photographs of Joseph Pilates himself, a barrel-chested ex-boxer with tattooed arms.

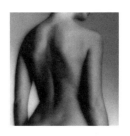

Born in Germany in 1880, Joseph was a sickly child who suffered from rickets, rheumatic fever and asthma. As if that wasn't tough enough, his parents clearly had it in for him and gave him the middle name Hubertus. This is now discretely shrunk to 'H' out of respect. Joseph was determined to overcome these handicaps and developed remarkable muscular control. He persisted with his self-development through gymnastics, diving and even working as a circus performer in England. In the spirit of fair play the English promptly rewarded him for this by interning him as a prisoner for the duration of World War I. Ever resourceful, he used the time to create his own exercise equipment with beds and bedsprings, devising exercise routines for his fellows and laying down the foundations of what he would call Contrology, and the rest of us call Pilates.

In the 1920s he emigrated to the US and opened a studio to teach physical fitness. Joseph's techniques became an instant hit with the dance world, which was quick to catch on to the Pilates' potential for healing injury while forging fine and firm physiques.

Joseph never stopped inventing ways of bringing exercise into daily life, and his exercises helped sculpt his own street-fighter shape as much as it toned the more elegant forms of his languid-limbed clientele. He wasn't one for wasting time as is shown both by his rewarding stint behind bars and the fact that he wooed his wife (and fitness studio partner) on board ship on his way to start a new life Stateside. Which is why I like to think he would have approved of this collection of ideas for variations on his exercises, and ways of working them into today's mad-dash lifestyle. History has associated the technique with dancers, with good reason, but the ideas in this book show that it has at least as much to offer to athletes, housewives and hairy-arsed builders with back trouble. I think Joseph would have been keen to spread the word to each and every one. Certainly I hope he would have approved – you wouldn't have wanted to pick a fight with the man.

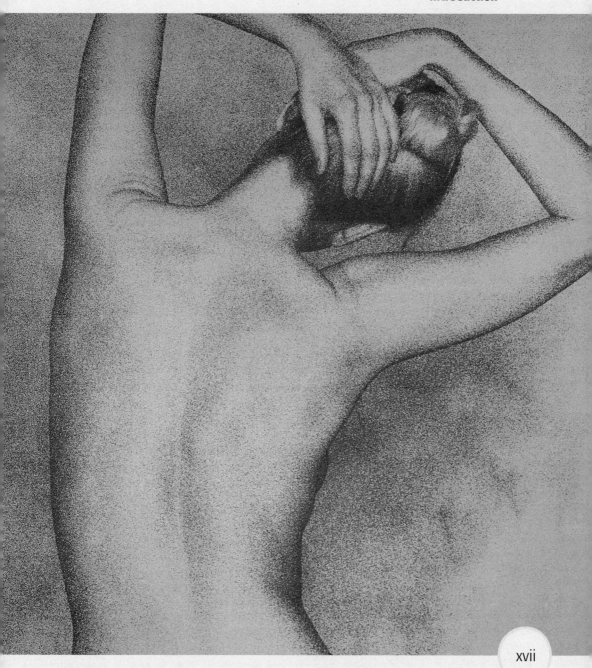

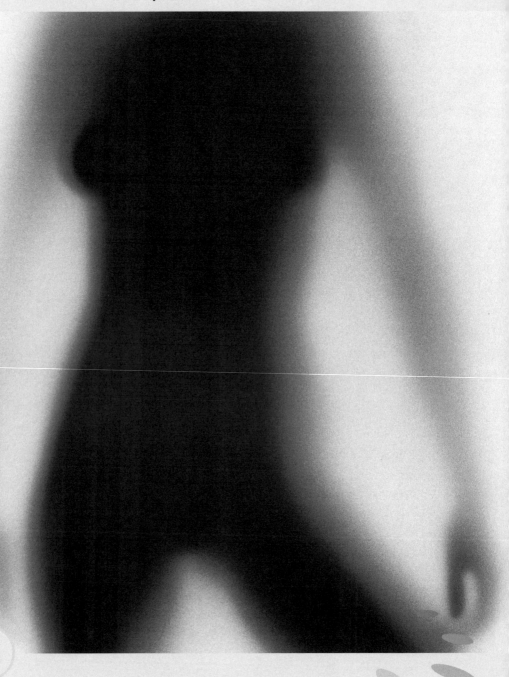

1

Back to basics

Joseph Pilates laid down eight basic principles which underlie all Pilates practice (and the ideas in this book). These are his brilliant ideas.

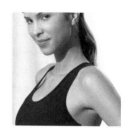

Actually the above is a lie. Joseph Pilates did lay down the principles of Pilates, but there's a catch.

The man may have mastered every muscle in his body but he clearly never got the hang of bullet points, lists or trademarks so there are a number of slightly different interpretations of what those eight were. In fact not everyone agrees on the number – some make it five, some six and there's at least one line of thought which trumps everyone else and manages to total nine. But these are the eight as I read them, and a few pointers on where to go next to work on each one.

1. CONTROL

When Joseph H. first pieced together his method he called it 'Contrology' and his most important work is called *Return to Life through Contrology*. 'Contrology' didn't stick (I always find it sounds a bit Orwellian) but it's worth noting how important was control to him. The concept of control in Pilates is about linking up the mind and body so that you have true body awareness. We tend to have some

Here's an idea for you... **Go back to point 1 above and this time rest your fingertips on the sides of your waist above the hips. Now try and tense the area where your fingers are. Feel it tense? OK, combine that with parking your pelvis (IDEA 6). You're starting to centre but there's more work to do. Now you've tensed that area, try to relax the front of your stomach. Relaxation is now being used as a concentration tool to help isolate the muscle at the side. When you manage to keep the side tense but the front relaxed (touch it with the other hand if that helps), then you only need to bring in the breathing element (breathe steadily, keep the muscle tense throughout) and you're well on the way to performing a muscle exercise Pilates style.**

mind/muscle controls well sorted out but others we just have to learn. Try this simple test. Without moving any part of your body tense your buttocks. Easy, right? Now tense your obliques (the muscles that run down the sides of your stomach and waist). You probably can't, or you tense the rectus abdominis (six-pack) at the front of the stomach. Pilates tries to establish mental control over the whole body, muscle by muscle.

2. BREATHING

Well, life would be a touch tricky without it but that doesn't mean we're doing it right. We use only a fraction of our lungs and often haven't developed the ability to breathe deeply with the diaphragm or 'widely' with the ribs. Take a look at IDEA 9, *A breath of fresh air*, for more.

3. FLUID MOVEMENT

There are exceptions where movement is fast (see IDEA 22, *Take that!*, or the jackknife in IDEA 52, *Topsy turvy II*) but even then the moves are controlled and fluid. This helps encourage grace but perhaps more importantly avoids the risk of injuring joints and losing muscular control over the exercise.

4. PRECISION

Pilates is very much about quality not quantity. There are very few repetitions and a lot of emphasis on getting it right, which is why instructions tend to be fairly detailed and include precise gestures and breathing.

While you're working with your waist, read a little more about what's going on under the skin (and padding) in IDEA 4, *Pants*.

Try another idea...

5. CENTRING

For some this is a reference to a Zen-like process of finding inner strength. Others mainly take it to mean the importance of neutral spinal alignment, and the core strength of the back and stomach that affects every other aspect of stability. For more, see IDEA 6, *Parking in neutral*.

6. STAMINA

Or 'routine' as some Pilates practitioners would have it. Routine doesn't mean doing the same thing every day and stamina doesn't mean doing the same thing over and over because this isn't the Pilates way. Instead it means getting into a regular pattern of exercise and enjoying workouts. For some, this could mean going to a studio three times a week, others might prefer practising Pilates moves in their daily life every day. See IDEA 8, *Post office Pilates*, and IDEA 10, *Are you sitting comfortably?*, for ideas on everyday Pilates.

7. RELAXATION

Different people come to Pilates for different reasons but one thing they all agree on is that unlike other workouts the Pilates approach

'Physical fitness is the first requisite of happiness.'
JOSEPH H. PILATES

Defining idea...

leaves you feeling refreshed and energised. Much of that is down to the careful way that the moves look to release stress that accumulates in the spine and the shoulders. For some instant stress-busters take a look at IDEA 11, *Pilates at the keyboard*.

8. CONCENTRATION

Relaxing doesn't mean letting it all go and Pilates is quite a mental workout. You have to focus on precisely what you are doing, often striving to isolate just one or two muscles; at other times you'll have to co-ordinate a host of them to work and balance at the same time.

How did it go?

Q   I'm not at all sure I can tense that side muscle at all. What can I do about that?

A   *Try working the obliques a little and then feeling for them. Take a look at the exercises in IDEA 26, Let's twist again. Eventually you'll make the bridge between mind and muscle.*

Q   I can't get the breathing right. Either I've completed the move before breathing out fully, or I have the opposite problem – I'm out of breath and racing to complete the move before I pass out. What should I do?

A   *For a start, don't hold your breath unless it's for a part of a move where your instructor expressly tells you to. It may take a little time, but if you're completing the move before you've breathed out fully you might want to think about slowing down a little. If you breathe out all the air before completing it, then breathe out less forcefully or accept that you need to start breathing in a little early until you have mastered the technique.*

2

Picking your Pilates instructor

The appeal of Pilates spans the spectrum from recovering rugby players to New Age mystics. Here's how to choose the flavour that's right for you.

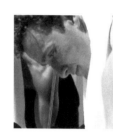

Pilates means many things to many people and a great deal of what is taught as Pilates today would have been completely new to Joseph H.

Back in 2002 the issue of what is and isn't Pilates was thrashed out in court as various factions bickered over who had the right to use the word. The result came as an irritation for Pilates purists who wanted to reserve the term for the teachings of Joseph H. himself. Instead it was decided that the term is generic, like 'yoga' or 'karate', and so people are free to use the term for any number of variations inspired by the original.

Some of the different flavours you may come across include:

■ **Authentic Pilates**™. Championed by The Pilates Guild™, this is Pilates the way Joe taught it personally, hence the 'authentic' tag. It's the pure, undiluted philosophy of the man himself, but doesn't include more recent developments such as Swiss ball work. Great for purists.

Here's an idea for you... If your gym has started Pilates classes or you happen to live next to a Pilates studio, then great. But it's more likely you'll have to look around a bit to find the type of Pilates you're after. The local papers or *Yellow Pages* may help you pin down a general Pilates practitioner, or you can search by UK region (as well as internationally) by visiting the Pilates Foundation website (www.pilatesfoundation.com). If you have more specific needs, such as recovering from injury or you're hoping to practice Pilates during pregnancy, then try www.pilates-world.com, which lists teachers with specialties.

■ **Contemporary Pilates**. This includes such well-known schools as Stott Pilates™ and Body Control Pilates™ which have updated some of the Pilates principles to include more recent thinking about posture and biomechanics. Joseph H. would often advise the 'locking' of joints like the knee in postures. That's now considered poor form in many activities, and isn't recommended in contemporary Pilates classes. This is the form of Pilates you're most likely to come across.

■ **Yogalates™/Yogilates**. This is a fusion of Pilates (which focuses on movements) and yoga (which focuses on holding positions) with the aim of increasing flexibility and reducing stress. The two spellings came about because Yogalates™ is trademarked and so many gyms or Pilates centres opt for the second spelling. Great for those looking for something a little different.

■ **PowerHouse Pilates**™. Part of a move to make Pilates more accessible to fitness instructors. Check out some of Lynne Robinson's books: she has shown that Pilates principles do translate to the modern gym. A fine way of combining good form, injury prevention and strength building.

■ **Winsor Pilates**™. Technique fusing Pilates and aerobics to increase fat burning and cardiovascular health. Bigger in the US than anywhere else, but some people swear by it to beat the bulge (see IDEA 12, *Weight loss with Winsor*).

It's not just the flavour of Pilates that varies but also the different ways of teaching. There are several approaches to both group and individual lessons – take a look at IDEA 3, *Class act*, to learn more.

Try another idea...

Plus there are a few other interesting variations such as Chi Pilates (another oriental fusion flavour), and a few euphemisms such as 'The Method' which are throwbacks to the days before the legal settlement when companies weren't sure about using the 'P' word.

Before you sign up for a course ask yourself just what you're after and ask the Pilates school exactly which kind of Pilates philosophy they follow. If you're more interested in the spiritual, then a combination of yoga and Pilates makes perfect sense. If, however, you're really interested in bench-pressing your own bodyweight and you've heard that Pilates can help you do it without popping a disc, then spending a lot of time in the 'resting child' position is unlikely to float your boat.

The degree of tuition of a Pilates instructor can vary from a couple of days to prepare them for a mat work qualification, to three or four years for a full and thorough qualification which will also take in the specialised Pilates equipment. If you think your Pilates trainer is expensive, or that there's another who looks like a bargain, then find out where they sit on the scale of qualifications.

'Variety's the very spice of life that gives it all its flavour.'
WILLIAM COWPER

Defining idea...

7

How did it go?

Q **My classes to date have been fine for grace and poise but we don't do a lot of strength work. What can I do if I want to work on strength?**

A *There are several options. You could ask your studio if they have resistance machines such as the Reformer (see IDEA 36, Rack and roll with the Reformer) and take tuition in those. Alternatively you can take your Pilates principles into the gym (see IDEA 18, Man and machine) or work on resistance at home (IDEA 31, Your flexible friend I).*

Q **I love the Pilates but I'm not losing the weight I want to. Is there any way I can combine Pilates and aerobics work?**

A *Winsor Pilates offers exactly that promise, and those who do Yogalates swear by it, but Joseph P was the first to fess up that Pilates isn't a total exercise programme and you might want to look at something a little more cardiovascular (swimming, running, walking, skipping) as well – remember you can still apply Pilates principles to other activities.*

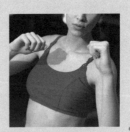

3

Class act

Still going to the same Pilates class every week? Worried that you've hit the Pilates plateau? Then try some different types of classes to break through that barrier and start making progress again.

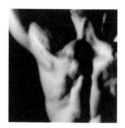

Pilates is based on the idea of a rich variety of exercises. Go to a class and you will never dwell on one exercise but instead be taken through a whole series of different approaches even if they work the same area of the body.

Go back to the same class the next day and you'll probably find yourself doing a completely different set again. That's no accident: the idea is that by constantly surprising the body with different ways of working we can be much more successful at making those essential mind to muscle links and perfecting our technique. Tedious repeated sets with hundreds of repetitions don't feature much and nothing is ever done to the point of fatigue. So why is it that so many people who practice Pilates don't think of applying the same approach to their class work? We are creatures of habit and whether we work out at home, take a private lesson or go to a class, the chances are that we stick to that same way of exercising week in, week out.

Here's an idea for you...

Pilates professionals will probably stone me for this but if you're not sure about coughing up £20 and upwards an hour, then start off with one of the videos or DVDs out there. A DVD player is by far the best because it's so much easier to freeze the frame and step forward and back without flickering spoiling the view. Plus the 'chapter' approach of DVDs makes it much faster to jump right back in where you left off.

WHAT'S OUT THERE?

Depending on which part of the country you happen to be in there'll be a variety of options. Not all of them can be found everywhere, but look around and you'll certainly find more than one choice that suits you.

GYM CLASSES

Depending on the facilities on offer these may be primarily mat based or may boast a complete Pilates suite with Cadillacs, Reformers, the lot. Not all gyms have the same approach to Pilates. Many offer basic mat work which is a great place to start and often included in your membership fee, but their instructors may not have the training to take it further. A few take it very seriously: the David Lloyd chain, for example, has linked up with Body Control Pilates™ to offer a very thorough and professional service.

Group mat class

This is the perfect place for beginners to start. It's relatively cheap, fun and sociable. More advanced practitioners often forget about group classes as they go on but because instructors all have their own ways of doing things there is often a lot to be learnt just by dipping into a different studio's group classes. Look out for a manageable student–teacher ratio of 10–15 students per class. Any more and the instructor won't be able to keep an eye on your technique.

Group Reformer class

Smaller, cheaper models of Reformer mean that quite a few studios and gyms are now offering Reformer classes. This is a great way to learn more about resistance work in Pilates with all the benefits of the group mat class.

Group ball class

Increasingly popular, not least because the equipment is cheap and they add a whole bunch of fun to the session.

Sessions for 2–4 students

Sometimes called duets, trios and quads, these small group sessions provide a compromise between the cost of private tuition and the attention of an individual session. For my money (of which there isn't a lot) they can provide the best value for the improver.

Private one-on-one session

Undoubtedly the best way to learn if you have the money and the time. If not, then it's worth saving up for the occasional treat because a single one-on-one session can help perfect the techniques that you will then take away into your home or *group* work.

Private one-on-one sessions with specialised equipment

If you want to get the hang of the Cadillac or Ladder Barrel, then this is often the only way as clubs and studios can rarely afford enough of these to offer group classes.

For more about what balls or Reformers could add to your Pilates regime, take a look at IDEA 29, *On the ball I*, and IDEA 36, *Rack and roll with the Reformer.*

Try another idea...

'*Life is a great school. It thrashes and bangs and teaches you.*'
NIKITA KHRUSHCHEV

Defining idea...

11

GETTING STARTED OR MOVING ON WITH A PILATES PROGRAMME

Mat work in group classes is the best way of getting to grips with Pilates. If you're not sure about what to expect, then you can always try videos or DVDs beforehand to get a feel for it. Moving on is a mix of varying your diet to take in different approaches (see above) and private tuition to perfect what you're practising. I really recommend trying some of the props (Swiss balls, bolsters, resistance bands, etc.) to bring something new to mat work at whatever level.

How did it go?

Q   **It's going great but I can't afford private tuition and I feel that I'm reaching the limits of the group classes I attend. Any ideas?**

A   *Yes. Find a studio that offers small classes (duets, trios, etc.) and round up some friends to make up your own group. Because the group is small it doesn't matter that you may have different levels of experience – the instructor should be able to get you doing your own thing and you will all contribute to keeping costs down.*

Q   **I'd love to have a go on the specialist machines but am skint. Do I have to bite the bullet and pay up for private tuition?**

A   *No, shop around and find a Pilates studio that offers classes using the newer, less expensive Reformers. Some gyms now offer this for six to eight people, each on their own Reformer and it makes for a much more reasonable way of trying out the hardware.*

4
Pants

Joseph H. Pilates liked to talk about the 'girdle of strength'. For those of us more used to the corset of corpulence here's how to craft your very own internal support underwear, and why a toned transversus beats a six-pack hands down.

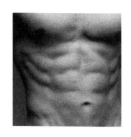

Stroll into a newsagent and take a look at the magazine covers. How many of them feature men and women clad in little more than a thong and a winning smile?

And of those, how many (women included) stomachs are so sculpted they seem to have internal scaffolding? It's the dreaded six-pack (or slab of chocolate if you're French), and our fascination with this quirk of anatomy has led loads of us to be mixed up and even thoroughly unhappy about our own bodies.

If an alien species were to research humanity on the basis of magazine covers it would decide we all had six-packs. If they were then to see the lot of us in the bathroom they'd be in for a surprise. A lot of Pilates books and articles (especially those in magazines with the rippled people on the cover) stress that it can help you develop strong stomach muscles and a toned tum. They're right. It can. Joseph H.

Here's an idea for you...

With the transversus we are aiming for toning – rather than build it any larger we simply want it to spend more time engaged and tight. The trick, therefore, is not just to rely on abdominal exercises but instead to try and tense the lower abdomen as often as you can remember to do so. Learn to make the effort whenever and wherever you are and you will build that girdle of strength.

was at great pains to explain the importance of a strong and toned midsection. What's often missed is that the first step towards that goal is to get rid of that fascination with the six-pack.

SLING THE SIX-PACK, GET TO GRIPS WITH GRIPPER KNICKERS

The six-pack is formed by a muscle called the rectus abdominis which runs up the front of your body from the ribs down to the pelvis. It's divided into different chunks as it goes down, which accounts for the six-pack effect, but the sharpness of that division (and even the number of chunks) is genetic. We can all make the rectus abdominis grow bigger and stronger but that doesn't mean we'll ever get the six-pack effect. Not unless grandpa and grandma were cover models.

But the rectus abdominis is only one of a team of muscles working to secure your stomach and flex your midriff. The others are the obliques and the transversus. The obliques run down the sides of your stomach and come into play when you twist or bend sideways. The transversus is the muscle that time, and magazine editors, forgot. It's a sheet of muscle that runs right across the front of your stomach from one side to the other. It lies underneath the limelight-hogging rectus so you'll never see it. What you can see, however, is the effect of a toned transversus. The transversus won't pump up as it strengthens, but instead it will develop muscle tone, meaning it will hold tighter at all times. Which in turn flattens the whole of your midsection, and gives you a longer, leaner look. It is nature's version of the 'control' pants ('gripper knickers') sold to try and tame tums that have an urge to expand beyond the limits of our clothes.

To work on toning the transversus rather than working the six-pack take a look at IDEA 5, *Scoop!*

Try another idea...

Six-packs are genetic. We don't all have the makings of a perfect six-pack but we all have a terrific transversus just itching to flatten out that midsection. Which is why so many of the Pilates moves require you to pull that navel in towards the spine, and up towards the ribs. As you do that you are building up that sheet of transversus muscle, with all the benefits that entails for posture, strength and of course looking fetching in swimwear.

Just one word of advice: no matter how good the results, no matter how tasty your tum turns out, the winning smile is fine, but the thong is never, ever, a good idea.

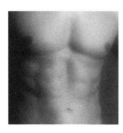

'You can only hold your stomach in for so many years.'
BURT REYNOLDS, on retiring from the big screen

Defining idea...

15

How did it go?

Q   **Are you sure I have abs at all?**

A   *Can you sit up in bed? Bend forwards? Lift your head and shoulders off the sofa when something interesting comes on the telly? Yes? Then you have abdominal muscles. They may not show (yet) because there's fat sitting there spoiling the view, but they're there and they're waiting to show you what they're made of.*

Q   **I'm tensing my stomach all right but I suspect I'm only sucking in the six-pack.**

A   *Explore a little. First rest your fingers on a point halfway from your belly to your naughty bits and try to tense at that point. Then put your fingers on your waist and try to tense there. Now try and tense these areas but simultaneously relax the front of your stomach beneath the ribs. As you learn about the different muscles you'll find it easier to disengage the six-pack which otherwise literally muscles in on the act.*

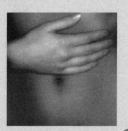

5

Scoop!

Whether your instructor calls it the 'B-line', the 'scoop' or 'zipping up', that Pilates toned tum is all about getting the pelvic floor and transversus muscles into play. You know that already because they keep telling you, but do you still wonder if you're doing it right?

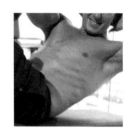

If you've read Idea 4, 'Pants', you'll know that the real secret to a toned tum isn't a bulging six-pack but a taut transversus. The next step is knowing just how to activate those deep internal muscles to protect your spine, improve your posture and, yes, look better in that bathing suit.

Every instructor has a different way of reminding you to engage those deep abdominal muscles, but if you find you're forever being told to 'zip up', 'scoop' or 'hollow' and you're still not completely sure of how to do it, then these are some tips from Pilates professionals around the planet.

One of the problems we often have with Pilates is losing the bad habits before we can pick up the new ones. After all, you've been sitting, standing and lying down for

Here's an idea for you...

When you're working on your Pilates exercises in the privacy of your own home, take the soft belt out of your dressing gown or towelling bath rope and just knot it loosely around your hips so it's on the B-line. Now do your Pilates routine and let the belt remind you to constantly tauten up from below the navel. Make sure it's a soft belt, loosely knotted. Try this with a belt with buckle and notches and you run the risk of doing yourself a mischief.

nearly all your life now without the benefit of someone telling you how, so it's no surprise that there's as much unlearning to do as learning. Because the rectus abdominis (six-pack) is a big, strong workhorse muscle, most of us leave it to do the work whenever we can. If we're told to pull in our stomachs, we do so from the front of our stomachs, trying to squeeze in rather than tense from the inside out. The problem for Pilates is that when we're told to adopt the classic position with 'navel to spine' most of us try and do that by using the rectus abdominis to squash our stomach in. It doesn't help that the 'navel to spine' line is a bit misleading – here's why.

B-line, or why navel gazing won't bring bellybutton and backbone together – try this:

Stand upright in the neutral posture – feet hip-width apart, knees very slightly bent, shoulders relaxed but not slumped. Now pull your stomach in as close to your spine as you can and breathe. There you go, navel to spine? Well maybe. But think for a moment about how your body feels, and answer these questions:

- Are your buttocks clenched?
- Does your breathing feel uncomfortable?
- Has your pelvis just tipped forward?
- Most of all, is the front edge of your ribcage now being pulled downwards?

The ribcage is the giveaway because if that has pulled down then it's because your rectus abdominis (six-pack) is doing the pulling. How unfair is that? You spend all your time bemoaning the fact that you can't see your six-pack only to find that you've got one after all and all it's doing is buggering up your perfect Pilates pose.

Still working on visualising those pelvic muscles? Then try IDEA 7, Workhorses and whippets.

Try another idea...

OK. Now try this:

Stand in neutral as before, feet hip-width apart, relaxed but not slumped. Draw a line with your fingers from one hip to the other across your tum. That's what some instructors call the 'B-Line'. Find the centre of that line ('B' marks the spot), it should be a couple of inches below your navel. Rest your finger on that spot and now try to pull the stomach in again but from that spot. Feel different? Feel as if you're working different muscles? Well you should be, and if you're contracting from that point, then all those other niggles (pelvic tilt/tipped ribcage/clenched bum) should melt away. That's the true posture, and the trick to remember that however much you're trying to pull navel to spine, the way to bring your backbone and bellybutton together is not to focus on the navel at all, but rather on a point a couple of inches below it.

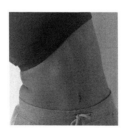

'He who does not mind his belly, will hardly mind anything else.'
SAMUEL JOHNSON

Defining idea...

THE SCOOP/ZIPPING UP

When instructors talk about 'scooping' or 'zipping up' they're referring to the same thing. The idea is not to hollow out your stomach by pulling in the front, but instead to start right deep in the pelvis and tighten up from there. Zipping is a visualisation technique to help you get there. Instead of sucking in that stomach, imagine instead that there's a zip running from the pelvic floor up to the ribs. Start to zip up from the very bottom and you should engage the pelvic muscles and the transversus rather than the abdominis.

How did it go?

Q   The B-line thing really helps, but our instructor tells us to zip up from the pelvic floor. How do I know where that is?

A   *If you're not sure where your pelvic muscles are, then just imagine that you're going for a pee. Just as you let fly you suddenly have to cut off that flow. Feel that tightening inside? There you go, that's where the muscles of your pelvic floor can be found.*

Q   I always start the move by scooping my stomach but can't keep it tight for long. What am I doing wrong?

A   *Can't keep it tight because you lose concentration or because you tire? If it's the latter, then just keep practising (see IDEA 8, Post office Pilates). If it's the former, then get in the habit of murmuring 'park and scoop' at the beginning and end of every pose to remind yourself until it becomes habit.*

6

Parking in neutral

Pilates instructors intone the words 'neutral position' like a sacred mantra and the whole class will duly pull their spines in or out a bit, but are you completely sure you know what it is?

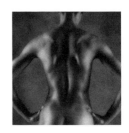

When I was younger I was forever being told to stand up straight. Come to think about it I was told to do a lot of things when I was younger, very few of which made much sense. When my teachers told me to stand up straight, however, they were doing me a favour. Well almost.

Joseph H. Pilates was not the first to notice the importance of proper posture for the body, but he did go a long way to pinning down exactly how it makes a difference, and he had the goodness to illustrate it for posterity with photos of himself showing bad posture. If you haven't seen those photos, then imagine a half-naked German indulging in the body language equivalent of gurning. Not pretty, but very educational.

Here's an idea for you... **Still struggling a little to find this neutral position? Try standing with your back against a wall so you can feel that surface. You are aiming to press as much of your back against the wall as possible. That doesn't mean standing ramrod straight. The gentle S-shape of the spine is an integral part of its design and some people have more of a curve than others. If you find that your back arches off the wall in the small of your back and you can't correct that with your pelvis in neutral, don't worry about it. Trying to make your spine straight up and down is not the point.**

That aside, stand upright, feet hip-width apart, knees slightly bent and slide your shoulder blades down your spine. You should be able to feel the wall between the blades. Experiment with angling the pelvis forwards and backwards and you will immediately feel how it pulls your back off the wall. Now try to set it in neutral and you should feel the maximum contact against your back.

One of the points he was making is that a misaligned spine is often down to the positioning of the pelvis and the muscles surrounding it. A pelvis that is tipped forwards or backwards will put pressure on the psoas muscles that run through it and connect the thigh to the spine. That in turn will help pull the spine one way or the other, leading to a lean forwards or backwards. While much of your body shape is genetic, a great deal of it comes from the way you stand.

As well as affecting posture, neutral positioning gives your body its most solid platform and thus its greatest strength. That reduces stress on all of the parts that link into the spinal column including joints, tendons and ligaments. Keeping your pelvis safely parked in neutral means you are working the way you were designed to do and that in turn helps minimise the chances of injury. Fitness instructors these days are taught to insist on neutral positioning for every single activity they do, but particularly for anything weight bearing. Neutral positioning can mean the difference between increased strength or being near crippled when weight lifting.

FINDING NEUTRAL

For more on posture take a look at IDEA 8, *Post office Pilates.*

Try another idea...

Lie on the floor flat on your back with your knees bent and your feet flat on the floor. Now place the heel of each hand on the projecting bones at the front of your pelvis. Touch your fingertips together at the top of the pubic bone (just by your pride and joy if you're a bloke) to form a triangle. This should be in a level plane, in fact one common visualisation trick is to imagine a glass of water balanced right there. Without using your legs at all use your stomach to push your lower back down towards the floor. This tilts the pelvis backwards and 'spills' the imaginary glass of water backwards towards your chest. Relax back to the neutral, middle, position, then try to tip your pelvis up the other way to spill the water again but in the opposite direction – this time it would spill between your legs. By deliberately taking the pelvis out of neutral and spilling that glass of water you can start to feel for the point when it's in neutral.

STANDING IN NEUTRAL

Now stand up and try to bring that knowledge to the upright position. Stand hip-width apart with your knees slightly bent and slide the shoulder blades down the spine. This is a standard stance for many upright activities. Imagine a string running up the middle of your spine and coming out of the top of your head, and think about being pulled up by that string as your neck extends. Now think about your pelvis and once again try to tip it as far forwards as you can, and then as far backwards. Since it is a little uncomfortable to have the pelvis in either of these positions, switching forwards and backwards between them should make it a blessed relief when you relax and return to the neutral point in between them.

'When the spine curves the entire body is thrown out of its natural alignment, off balance.'
JOSEPH H. PILATES

Defining idea...

Q   **I'm looking in the mirror and think I've got this neutral thing cracked. Anything I might have missed?**

A   *Are you standing face on. Of course you are, who doesn't. Turn sideways and while squinting furiously out of the side of your eyes check that your ears, shoulders, hips, knees and ankles are aligned as if an overzealous architect had hung a plumb line on you from the ears right down to the feet.*

Q   **When I'm in neutral flat on my back I can slide a hand under the small of my back but I don't feel like I'm arching. Am I doing something wrong?**

A   *Not necessarily. We all have a different amount of curve in our spine and the idea is not to try and flatten it out unnaturally. Don't focus on the small of your back and just concentrate on tipping your pelvis forwards and backwards until you're sure you're in neutral.*

7

Workhorses and whippets

Pilates isn't just about tight tums and long legs (though that would be enough for most of us), it's about achieving balance through a better understanding of the muscles of our body.

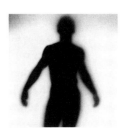

On the face of it there's not a lot of similarity between the worlds of pumped-up bodybuilders and long, lean Pilates practitioners, but although they probably don't know it there's one important belief they share.

Ask a bodybuilder whether they prefer free weights (dumbbells and barbells) or machine weights and they'll let you know in no uncertain terms that free weights are vastly superior for building muscle. Ask them why and they'll point to things like range of movement, and the important role played by stabiliser muscles in balancing a large weight held in the hands. They may also offer to demonstrate but that's the time to make your excuses and leave.

The point is that even the meatheads realise that true strength rarely comes from just building up the 'show' muscles like the biceps of the arms or pectorals of the chest. There is a network of minor muscles that are recruited to help out with every

*Here's an
idea for
you...*

Let your fingers do the walking. Often in classes you'll be told to perform a technique in such a way so as to isolate a muscle and work it, rather than the workhorse that will otherwise do the job. Try where possible to touch that muscle with your fingers to get a feel for it – you'll find it much easier to visualise it and make that mind–body connection. For example, try contracting your tricep muscle (the back of your arms) without bending your elbow at all. Now touch the back of your arms with the other hand and try again so you can feel the muscle. You should find it much easier to contract it and understand where it starts and stops.

job of work and for all-round strength it's important to get them all in on the act.

Leaving those pumped-up guys in cut-off vests behind for a moment, and entering the Zen-like calm of a Pilates studio you might think you're in a totally different world. In fact one key part of the body philosophy is the same in both – that true strength comes from working all of the minor muscles. The key difference is that the bodybuilders are only hitting the minor keys as a supporting act for their show muscles. In Pilates the focus is on redressing the body imbalance by trying to leave the big workhorse muscles out of it altogether, and exercising those smaller, lighter, secondary muscles. It's about workhorses and whippets, and when you enter the Pilates studio you should be trying to give the workhorses a break, and let the whippets work up a sweat. That's why so many Pilates exercises don't involve large, strong movements that would work the big muscles, and it's also why there's so much focus on technique to ensure your body isn't cheating and letting the big boys do all the work.

GETTING TO KNOW YOU, GETTING TO KNOW ALL ABOUT YOU

Most of us have a fair idea of the muscles down our fronts but are usually a bit less familiar with those in our backs. That's normal since short of peering round our shoulders in a mirror we don't get to see our backs much. Try getting to know the muscles in your back and shoulders and see how to relax the workhorses and let the whippets play.

For an example of isolating a muscle that is normally helped out by workhorses take a look at IDEA 48, *Forearm smash*.

Try another idea...

Lie on the floor face down with your arms down by your sides, relaxed. Now smoothly, and without using your arms, lift your head and chest off the floor so you arch upwards. Don't worry about lifting up too high, and if you feel back pain, then stop. Keep your eyes facing the floor as you perform the movement. Imagine you have an apple tucked between your chin and your throat and try to keep it held there. Try to think about the muscles you're using.

That's an exercise called a back extension. It works the erector spinae muscles which run all the way down the centre of your back and which you use to arch backwards. Think of these spinal erectors as the equals and opposites of the famous six-pack that pulls your ribcage forwards as you bend. Now, try the same move again but with your arms out in front of you, bent at the elbows, a little as if you were at the start of a breaststroke arm movement only with the palms facing the floor. Now pull both shoulders back together so the elbows go right back as if they were going to bump into your ribcage. Feel those muscles. You should feel the movement in two big triangular muscles that run from between your shoulder blades right out to your shoulders and down towards your bum in a big V-shape. Those are your laterals ('lats').

'There is another important reason for consistently exercising all our muscles: namely that each muscle may cooperatively and loyally aid in the uniform of all our muscles. Developing minor muscles naturally helps to strengthen major muscles. As small bricks are employed to build large building so will the development of small muscles help develop large muscles.'
JOSEPH H. PILATES

Defining idea...

Back extensions and lateral flexions are great exercises but they are not Pilates exercises. Pilates works on trying to isolate the smaller muscles of control and balance.

Now try lying on the floor face down as before. Zip up (see IDEA 5, *Scoop!*) and slide your shoulder blades down into your back, lifting your face off the floor lightly but not by arching your back – imagine instead that your neck is growing longer and longer and try to extend your spine forwards as you slide your shoulder blades backwards. Feel the muscles you're using now. Different? They should be. If you're sliding your shoulders down and back and lengthening your neck, then you should manage to avoid the lats and instead be gently working the lower trapezius (more commonly used when we shrug) and the serratus muscles that attach to the backs of the ribs.

Recognising those subtle differences in movement that recruit totally different muscle groups is part of the art of Pilates.

How did it go?

Q   I tried the front-down floor exercise, but how come when I try to feel my muscles all I feel is strain at the top of my neck?

A   *Make sure you're not lifting the head high or looking down so the neck is out of line with the spine. Concentrate on extending it outwards as if it was growing like Pinocchio's nose.*

Q   I'm trying to relax the erector spinae but I can still feel them stiffening all the way down my spine. What am I doing wrong?

A   *Make sure you're not trying to lift your chest too high, and keep your feet firmly on the floor – if they lift up, then you are trying to curl your body like a bow which will mean your spinal muscles are pulling your pelvis upwards.*

8

Post office Pilates

The Full Monty showed us how queuing should really be done – twirls, hip thrusts and all – but for those of us who don't have the moves or the music there are other ways of playing the waiting game to win.

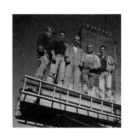

You will spend five years of your life standing in line. That's not including all that time on the bus/tube spent glaring at the youth of today in the hope that one of them will crack and offer you his seat.

In Britain queuing is the unofficial national sport. It's being proposed as a relay event to the Olympic Committee and the discipline of First-day-of-the-sales Full Contact Queuing may soon be recognised as a formal martial art. In the meantime you might as well use some of that time on your feet to keep your body on its toes, as it were.

It doesn't matter if you're standing in line for stamps, waiting for a bus or queuing for the border at Burkina Faso, you can always use the time to check your neutral stance and tone your torso.

Here's an idea for you...

Many of us struggle with our stomach muscles (presuming we can find any) and years of sucking the stomach in at the swimming pool do little to train us for a perfectly toned tum. To help you maintain that taut but elastic approach try two things:

■ **Don't focus on the rectus abdominis (or 'abs') that make up the six-pack we all see in the magazines. Think instead of the transversus abdominis, the sheet of muscle that lies underneath the abs. To know more about how the transversus works, take a look at IDEA 4, *Pants*. Instead of seeking to scrunch up your six-pack, think about tensing your transversus.**

■ **Lightly place the tips of your fingers between your navel and your knickers as you breath. Feel the navel being pulled in and the tautness of your abdominal muscles as they rise and fall with the incoming breath.**

First make sure you're standing with your feet hip-width apart, facing directly forward, knees very slightly bent and your shoulders nice and relaxed but not slumped. Check that your pelvis is in neutral (see IDEA 6, *Parking in neutral*) by tilting it forwards and backwards until you find the midpoint. If you genuinely are in line for an immigration official, police checkpoint or anything at all when in prison, then it's best not to rock your pelvis forward and back too vigorously. You might be sending out the wrong signals.

Without bending your neck forwards, tilt your head so that your chin drops very slightly forward to extend the neck and help elongate the spine.

Breathe deeply. Really deeply, right down into your lower abdomen. Time to contemplate your navel. Focusing on your belly button, use your abdominal muscles to pull it right in towards your spine and up towards your ribs. Keep breathing in deep into the abdomen – it may seem a little strange at first but you should be able to do this without relaxing your stomach muscles. The aim is not to have your stomach clenched like a fist, but instead taut and elastic so that it is flattened but still rises as you draw air into your body.

Now breathe into your stomach, and gently out again for ten long, slow breaths. Of course you don't actually breathe into your stomach, but that's how it should feel. (For more on that subject see IDEA 9, *A breath of fresh air.*)

Concentrate on that stomach, on keeping your shoulders relaxed, and on emptying all the air out of your lungs as you breath out.

As well as practising your Pilates stance, toning your tum and taking your mind off the wait, this should also help calm you down and reduce your stress levels. Perfect for when the muppet at the front of the queue walks up to the counter and asks for 'six first-class stamps...and a complete change of name and nationality, please'.

Tube stuck in the tunnel? Bus bogged down by roadworks? Bored witless and don't care who knows it? Then move on to some standing stretches while you're there – if nothing else it will keep the rest of the queue/bus/train entertained – see IDEA 27, *Lateral thinking.*

Try another idea...

'Standing also is very important and should be practiced at all times until it is mastered.'
JOSEPH H. PILATES

Defining idea...

31

How did it go?

Q   **I can hear a noise in my throat as I inhale – is that right?**

A   *Sounds like you've dropped your chin too far and are constricting the airways of the throat. While tilting the head forward is a great way of extending the spine it shouldn't go so far that it interferes with breathing.*

Q   **I'm what they call 'generously proportioned' and when I rest my fingertips beneath my navel I don't feel anything tense. Am I doing it wrong?**

A   *Not necessarily no. Most of us have a little padding between our stomach muscles and the outside world and sometimes this is generous enough so that we feel the fat, not the muscle, on our tums. Instead of feeling for the muscle with your fingers, just feel for the rise and fall as you try to pull air into your lower body rather than your upper chest. Independently of that, try and sense the internal contraction right across the front of your body from one side to the other as the sheet of muscle contracts.*

9

A breath of fresh air

Breathing properly is something we take for granted – after all, if you were doing it wrong you'd be dead, right? Which is why it may come as a surprise to find that breathing better is one of the fundamental Pilates principles.

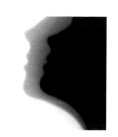

Professional singers will tell you that the voice comes from the diaphragm, not from the throat, and Pilates breathing follows much the same principal.

It's often referred to as breathing from the belly because it feels as if you are drawing air right down into your guts. Of course that's not the case: you breathe with your lungs, which will hopefully spend the whole of your life locked firmly away in the ribcage. There is more to breathing, however, than the rise and fall of that ribcage.

Small muscles called the intercostals stretch from rib to rib and expand the chest by pulling the ribs apart, which in turn draws air into the lungs. If you want to see the astonishing power of the intercostals, then all you have to do is line up a group of flabby, middle-aged men at a swimming pool and wait until a bikini-babe walks by.

Trying to imagine breathing 'wide' rather than deep is often a bit tricky, so let your fingers help you understand. Place your hands behind you, palms on the sides of your back as high up the ribcage as is comfortable. Now breathe in and feel the expansion of the ribs to the sides. When you breathe normally the sides will barely move, if at all. Try to breathe into the sides of your ribcage, making them expand outwards as much as possible. Feel how you draw the air in with a muscular effort of the chest to the sides, rather than simply swelling the chest out to the front. Breathe in steadily through the nose for five seconds, then exhale through the mouth for the same count.

Those suddenly swelling chests are all down to intercostals. Oh, and male vanity of course. Some Pilates teachers refer to the idea of breathing 'wide'. Instead of breathing 'deeply,' they will say breathe 'widely' and that means trying to get the most out of the intercostals. We tend to think of breathing in the chest as being a forwards and backwards movement, but in fact our ribcage can extend to the sides as well. To breath widely, think about filling your lungs so much that you can feel your shoulder blades being pulled gently apart as your sides expand.

The other muscle that affects the way we breathe is the diaphragm, a sheet of muscle below the lungs that divides our chest from our abdomen. When the abdomen contracts it pushes down into the abdomen and that fills our lungs with air. Imagine a doctor filling a hypodermic syringe from a bottle that they're holding up to the light. The syringe is the lung, the plunger is the diaphragm. As the plunger is pulled down it sucks the liquid out of the bottle into the syringe. As the diaphragm pushes down into the abdomen it sucks the air down the windpipe and into the lungs.

The more the plunger is pulled down, the more liquid is sucked in – same with the diaphragm drawing air into the lungs, and that's what 'belly breathing' is all about. It's not really air you feel being drawn into your stomach, it's the effect of the diaphragm compressing your abdomen. Ignore that detail though, and instead imagine that you are sucking the air in right down to your navel.

Now you've cracked this breathing thing, it's time to learn how to stand up – see IDEA 8, *Post office Pilates*. Honestly, we'll be telling you how to sit down next...

Try another idea...

Most of the time we breathe quite shallowly, using only about a quarter of our true lung capacity. Pilates teachers often refer to that as breathing into the top of the chest. By belly breathing we use much more of the lung capacity, as well as working the abdominal muscles that give us core strength.

Never try to hold your breath in Pilates: breathing, just like every other movement, should always be smooth and continuous. If you're unsure about when to breathe in or out, the general rule is that you exhale as you perform the action and inhale on the recovery. If you've misjudged your breathing and run out of breath to exhale before finishing the move, then take another breath. You might not think you need to be told when to breathe, but in practice most of us are tempted to hold our breath as we concentrate on finishing the move.

'Above all learn how to breathe correctly. Squeeze every atom of air from your lungs until they are almost as free of air as is a vacuum.' JOSEPH H. PILATES, clearly enjoying a little head spin from time to time

Defining idea...

35

How did it go?

Q   I get dizzy. Am I meant to?

A   *No. Despite Joseph Pilates' exhortation to squeeze all the air out of your lungs, this is best read as an encouragement to breathe deeply to flush the lungs out. If you aren't used to such deep breathing and you force all the air out you may well get dizzy, and however much fun that was when we were kids it won't help with your concentration.*

Q   I have stomach, yes, plenty of it thanks. Whether I am breathing with it is hard to say. Any tips?

A   *Again let your own fingers help tell you what's happening down there. Rest your fingers on your lower abs between the belly button and the naughty bits and try to breathe into that lower belly. In reality it's not your belly that's breathing (unless you are very unusual) but with practice it will feel as if your belly is sucking the breath right down to your navel.*

10

Are you sitting comfortably?

Pilates isn't just about classes or mat work. Its principles can be applied to almost any situation, making it possible to do yourself some good wherever you are – in the office, on the bus or down the pub.

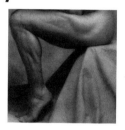

Life, I find, has an irritating habit of butting into my schedule of exercise and well-being. In theory I have an eight-hour regime of taking care of myself in the gym and Pilates studio, but in practice little things like work, family and friends tend to get in the way.

One of the beauties of Pilates is that it can be applied to almost any physical activity – or inactivity. You can be working out without anyone knowing. You really can be working out by sitting on your arse.

Sitting isn't as easy as it looks. Most of us manage to put stress on our shoulders, necks and backs just by the way we sit. Pilates posture can help.

Here's an idea for you...

'The lift' is another exercise you can do at your office chair or on the bus. The aim is to work on zipping up from the bottom of the pelvis towards your ribs. While sitting upright, imagine that there is a lift on your pelvic floor. As you breathe out try to take that lift 'up' to the next floor – you should feel your pelvic muscles go taut. As you take the 'lift' further up the floors from 'first' to 'second', you should feel your lower abdominals tighten. Higher than that and you risk the six-pack muscling in on the action. If you're not sure why that's such a bad thing, then turn to IDEA 5, *Scoop!*

First, make sure you're sitting back in your chair with your feet flat on the floor. Imagine that your coccyx (tailbone) is made of lead and pulling straight down into the chair. Make sure your spine is in neutral and you can feel the middle of your back lightly pressed against the seat back. Your shoulders should be relaxed but not slumped. Feel for the B-line and zip up (see IDEA 5, *Scoop!*). To get a feel for that position try some leg lifts. Lift each knee alternately up, placing it smoothly down again with the foot flat on the floor. You should be totally stable, if you can feel your coccyx moving, then check that you are sitting back and in the neutral position – you may be sitting too far forward with your pelvis tilted. If you're not sure about neutral when sitting, then try lifting the knee right up towards your chest. As you do you'll reach a point where you can feel the pelvis tilt, and the coccyx slides towards the front of the seat. Hopefully that feel for being out of neutral should help you settle into neutral.

With your pelvis and back sorted out, the next issue is your shoulders and the neck strain that all too easily results from tension and poor posture. Hunching your shoulders upwards is a shortcut to tension and trouble as it tightens the trapezius muscle at the top of your back and that transmits its strain into the back of the neck. If you feel tense (and who doesn't at some point in the working day) then try this.

Slide your shoulder blades towards each other and then down and at the same time extend your neck. You should feel an immediate easing of the pressure on your spinal column, shoulders and neck as well as feeling as if you've just grown an inch. Next time you want to shout at someone, try doing that first.

'The greatest monarch on the proudest throne is obliged to sit upon his own arse.'
BENJAMIN FRANKLIN

Defining idea...

A really great time to try the sitting exercises is on the bus/tube or at the traffic lights on the way home. Because we're tired we're likely to slump and take all that tension back home with us. Try and make it part of your daily routine to ease that pressure out as a way of leaving work behind before you get home. Don't forget that it's just as effective in the pub or sat in front of *Friends*.

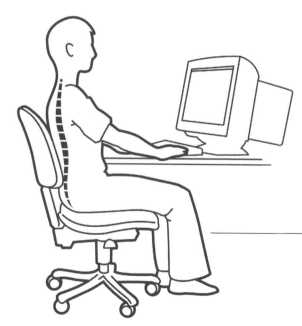

You'll find more hints to beat the slouch in IDEA 11, *Pilates at the keyboard,*

Try another idea...

Are you sitting comfortably?
Scoop that stomach, park that pelvis and we'll begin.

How did it go?

Q **When I sit down I find my lower spine arches away from the back of the chair. What am I doing wrong?**

A *Check your shoulders. Are you pulling them back as on a military inspection? Relax your shoulders without dropping them, and if that doesn't do it check you're not tilting your pelvis backwards. If you're sporting rather a lot of extra curves on the tum this may pull your middle forwards and tilt your pelvis.*

Q **I set myself up in the right position but after a while I notice that I've inevitably slipped back into my habitual hunched slouch – keeping it up is as hard as it was at school when we were told to sit upright. Any ideas?**

A *Know just what you mean. It takes time to get rid of bad habits and the problem is made worse because unless you have a very unusual job you're probably not just sitting there – you're probably reaching for the phone and keyboard too. It will come and it will feel more comfortable but at first just try and set yourself a series of breaks – maybe every twenty minutes or half hour – and try the exercises in IDEA 11, Pilates at the keyboard, then 're-set' your sitting position and off you go again. In time you will feel easier sitting in neutral than you did in your old slump.*

11
Pilates at the keyboard

Pilates is a great way of avoiding injury and you don't have to be a dancer to benefit – the average desk jockey risks quite enough damage at work, and a few simple moves can ease the pain of the working day.

Pilates first found fame as a way for injured dancers to recover their strength and mobility. With its emphasis on building up tone with low stress and few repetitions it proved a great way of recovering dynamically — essential for those aiming to get back to full fitness as fast as possible.

These days the walking wounded that turn to it are just as likely to be office workers with back pain and stiff necks. Ironically many of them will perform their Pilates moves with great care and attention in the studio, then go back to doing exactly what caused the problem once they're back in the familiar surroundings of the office. While the studio is undoubtedly the place to learn new moves, you can

Put your arm up in the air, bend your elbow and allow your hand to rest on the top of your head with your fingers on the side just touching your ear. Now gently ease into a stretch by pulling very lightly with the hand while resisting gently with the head and neck muscles as if you were trying to straighten your neck against the pull of your hand. Don't overdo it: this is a gentle release of the muscles in the neck for just a few seconds. Now reverse arms and do the other side. Now roll your head back and circle. There, feel slightly less homicidal now?

practice them just about anywhere on the planet, and Pilates in the office is a great way of preventing those problems from showing up in the first place. Take it from me. I found out the hard way. A professional life slaving over a hot keyboard left me with chronic back pain, stiff hands and an amusingly lop-sided neck from clutching a phone under my chin. These days I make sure I get away from the keyboard often enough to give my body a break, but when deadlines are tight, or the boss is hanging over your shoulder, you don't have to leave your seat to perform simple exercises to release those muscles, help your posture and above all ease the stress.

Since we tend to store up stress in the shoulders, try to roll it out again with shoulder rotations. Mobility exercises – taking the joints through their full range of movement – are a staple of most forms of modern exercising and Joseph H. was a great fan as can be seen from exercises like the one leg circle which was one of the first he taught in *Return to Life through Contrology*. Your shoulder, like your hip, is a ball and socket joint, meaning it can rotate in any direction, so every now and again you should let it. Sitting in neutral, with your feet flat on the floor and your shoulders relaxed but not slumped, bend your elbows and rest your fingertips on your shoulder (right on right, left on left). Now circle them forwards and upwards so your elbows touch, then lift up above your ears, pull back to be in line with your shoulders and finally come forward again. Now perform the same circle but in the opposite direction – remember the importance of working every equal and opposite muscle so that for every pull there is a push.

Spend a lot of time sat down? Take a look at IDEA 10, *Are you sitting comfortably?*

Try another idea...

The best office destressing exercise is undoubtedly to land a clean right hook on the boss, but since this may lead to ugliness it's worth looking at other options. Stress balls – those squidgy balls you can squash in your fist when anxiety rises – are a good exercise for your hand muscles. The problem is people often tense the trapezius muscle that leads to the shoulders when they do. If you use a stress ball, then make sure you perform the shoulder roll above.

Now work on the fingers – if you've been typing, then they're probably tense and tired. Despite the publicity about RSI you only have to look around any office for a couple of minutes and you'll find keyboards without wrist wrests, keyboards set up at the wrong height for the seat and keyboards right at the edge of the desk so there's nowhere to rest your elbows. Concentrated mouse work, even with elegantly shaped ergonomic mice, can also put real pressure on your fingers. Remember that before you start your fiftieth game of minesweeper.

'To neglect one's body for any other advantage in life is the greatest of follies.'
SCHOPENHAUER, as quoted by Joseph H. Pilates

Defining idea...

To release tension in the fingers start by turning your hands palm upwards and bring the tip of each finger in turn to the tip of your thumb then repeat the sequence. Just to make things a little more interesting, try starting with the little finger on one hand at the same time as you start at the index finger on the other so the two hands are out of synch.

Next, hold all your fingers our flat together and then open up the gap between the second and third fingers so that the first and second pull away in one direction and the third and fourth in the other. Sci-fi fans will immediately recognise this as the Vulcan greeting. Now bring the second and third fingers together and keep them together and this time open up the gaps between the first and second, and third and fourth. Try not to do this if the self-appointed office wit is around, otherwise Spock/Mork and Mindy gags will follow you around forever.

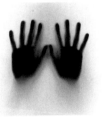 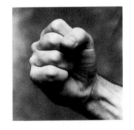

Q   **When I do the shoulder roll and stretch my shoulder blades back, why does my neck go tense?**

How did it go?

A   *The aim is to move the shoulders rather than the shoulder blades. If you concentrate on keeping the middle of your upper back (the bit between the shoulder blades) in contact with the chair you should isolate the movement of the shoulder itself.*

Q   **I can't do that 'Vulcan' thing – I'm not sure my fingers work that way.**

A   *Then try playing an imaginary piano instead. Then turn your palms up the other way and try playing an imaginary upside-down piano (who says you don't get to have fun in the office?).*

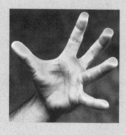

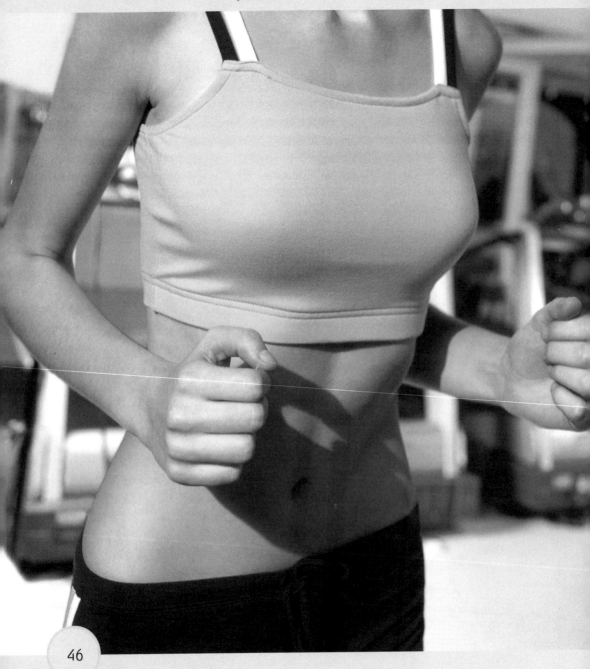

12

Weight loss with Winsor

Even Joseph H. Pilates never claimed that his exercises were enough to make you completely fit. Winsor Pilates, on the other hand, claims that it does.

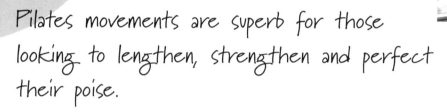

Pilates movements are superb for those looking to lengthen, strengthen and perfect their poise.

What they don't offer, however, is a meaningful cardiovascular workout. If it's calorie burning you're after, then the low repetition, smooth, studied movements of Pilates are not enough to increase your metabolism and burn off the fat. Just the opposite in fact. In *Return to Life through Contrology* Joseph H. wrote that 'Contrology exercises guard against unnecessary pounding or throbbing of the heart...all the exercises are performed while you are in a sitting or reclining position. This is done to relieve your heart from undue strain.'

Contemporary Pilates has added standing movements to the classic Contrology canon, but in general the point about the heart rate remains true today.

As the importance of aerobic exercise has become evident, and jogging, aerobics, rollerblading and their like have come and gone as the fitness fad of the moment, there have been a number of attempts to inject a cardiovascular element into

Most people who try Winsor Pilates seem to speak highly of it but just about everyone mentions the cost. So if you're interested but hesitating, then try and rent it. If you can't find it in your local video shop, then why not buy second hand? Take a look at online auctioneer eBay (www.ebay.com) and you'll find plenty of copies of the Winsor video for sale, along with all the other fitness equipment that gets used and then collects dust. Buy it second hand, give it a whirl and then sell it on again when you're done with learning from it.

'It would be a grave error to assume that even Contrology exercises alone will remake a man or a woman into an entirely physically fit person.'
JOSEPH H. PILATES

Pilates. Sometimes these are just a little token, as for example those Swiss ball classes that attempt to up your heart rate by bouncing for a few minutes. True it does speed up your metabolic rate, but it simply won't account for that dollop of Chantilly crème, let alone the extra large serving of chocolate mousse it happened to adorn.

CUE WINSOR PILATES

Heavily hyped through infomercials on US TV, Mari Winsor's approach has been to take moves based on Pilates principles of joint mobility, neutral positioning and core strength, and combine them in what she calls 'dynamic sequencing'. This isn't aerobics and avoids both pumping backbeats and high-impact work. Workouts range from a 20 minute shorty, to a 50 minute fat burner, and true to Pilates form it moves swiftly on from one exercise to the next so you have little chance to get bored (unless it's with the voiceover).

There are some undoubted negatives though. It's expensive (make no mistake, that Mari Winsor runs a mean marketing machine), and it doesn't take the heart rate up as high as aerobic sessions, nor does it do much for your arms or chest. In the States it's heavily endorsed by celebrities and in particular the two 'faces' of Winsor are Daisy Fuentes and Elizabeth Berkeley. The first is a Latina model, and the latter an actress best known for stripping off in the film *Showgirls.* You only have to look at pictures of the pair of them through their careers (and believe me I have) to realise that neither has exactly been battling a weight problem so I'm stuck as to how they demonstrate the benefits of the system, but hey, what do I know?

If you're interested in fat burning but refuse point blank to strap on running shoes or set foot in an aerobics studio, then Winsor Pilates may be your bag. If you're a Pilates purist, on the other hand, then you may want to avoid the videos in case it provokes apoplectic seizure.

Try another idea...

There are no cardiovascular moves in Pilates but if you're interested in calorie burning you may want to bear in mind that strength training also raises metabolism. Muscle simply demands a lot more maintenance than fat and a more muscular person will, pound for pound, use up more calories simply by sitting down than their less muscular mates. So take a look at some of the ideas on resistance work, such as IDEAS 16 and 17, *Getting smart with dumbbells I and II.*

Defining idea...

'*Working with Mari Winsor and the Pilates technique has proven to be the absolute best workout for my body, mind, and soul.*'
ELIZABETH BERKELEY

How did it go?

Q **What's a 'tushie'?**

A *Ah, did I forget to mention that? It seems that Ms Winsor has some obscure grudge against the word 'buttocks' and for some reason thinks that the word 'tushie' is more acceptable. Personally I feel that's a bunch of arse but that may be some kind of gender/culture gap and anyway I suspect that I'm not the target market. Just ignore it and watch the pictures.*

Q **I'm mostly interested in warding off osteoporosis. Winsor mainly seems to be about losing weight. Will it still help me?**

A *Yes, Winsor is effectively a low-impact aerobic workout. What that means is that compared to high impact (like running or step class) it avoids a lot of the shock of your body hitting the ground. It still involves moving your weight from foot to foot and carrying your own body mass so it will help increase bone density.*

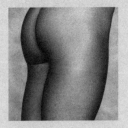

13

This little piggy does Pilates

Next time you put your feet up don't just give them a break – give them a workout.

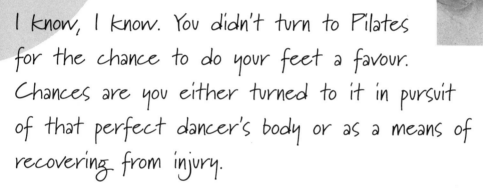

I know, I know. You didn't turn to Pilates for the chance to do your feet a favour. Chances are you either turned to it in pursuit of that perfect dancer's body or as a means of recovering from injury.

Feet did not come into the equation. Like most adults you tend to hide your feet away and if we're going to be brutally honest you probably consider them a bit ugly. Time to change all that and for two very good reasons:

- You don't have to be a reflexologist to realise that the feet hold the key to easing stress and keeping the rest of the body happy.

- You might not think it as you apply that corn plaster, but the feet themselves are a miracle of anatomical engineering and deserve the best maintenance you can give them.

Try playing imaginary piano scales with your toes (you'll need to be barefoot for this). Joseph H. Pilates was a great believer in body control and this is a great exercise for trying to re-establish the links between brain and body. With the soles of your feet flat on the ground, spread your toes as wide apart from each other as you can and then try to touch them to the ground one after another in order. It's not as easy as you might think. Remember they have to touch one at a time and in order. Got that? No problem? OK, then I'll bet you just did it starting with the little toe. Now try to reverse that and do it the other way, starting with the big toes.

The first point is easy to prove. Next time you get back home from the shopping trip or from work, kick your shoes off, lose those socks/fishnets and with your bare foot just try to grip the carpet, then relax. Doesn't that feel good? Doesn't that feel good right through to your shoulders? In fact it feels so good you should do it right now. I don't care if you're in the office, tell the boss I said it was OK. We all know that daily stress makes its way into the shoulders, and while I'm not knocking the divine beauty that is the back rub, if you forget about your feet, then you're only dealing with the most obvious symptom of stress.

Your feet contain 52 bones, and more than 76 muscles and ligaments. More than a quarter of all the body's bones are in the feet, most of them are small and delicate, and yet everyday we expect them to handle the equivalent of hundreds of tons of force with barely a thought for their well-being.

Trust me, I'm a runner, which means I've done more than my fair share of foot abuse without a thought for any of the above. Until the day when something goes wrong of course. Once you've picked up a foot injury you start to realise how tough life is when walking becomes a problem, so take care of those feet.

A foot workout doesn't have to take long and will go a long way to easing stress. As ever, even though you're thinking of your toes you shouldn't neglect your posture. As you sit, park your pelvis in neutral, and pull your head and spine upright as if being pulled up by a string running right through your spine and out through the top of your head. Scoop your stomach and now focus on your feet.

Start with a little ankle rotation to ease swelling and increase mobility. Rotate each foot in a circle while keeping the knee and lower leg still. Now try rotating them both together but in opposite directions and then change direction to circle the other way. If you've been walking all day, and especially if you've been carrying heavy bags, then this should ease the pressure immediately.

Now try pointing and flexing both feet together. Pointing means pushing your toes as far away from you as you can but try not to curl the toes, instead keep them straight and in line with the foot. Flexing means turning the ankle the other way so that the toes point back towards you, again the toes should be in line with the foot rather than trying to bend right back.

Enjoying the footwork? Fancy some more exercises you can do behind the desk? Then take a look at IDEA 14, *Playing footsie*.

Try another idea...

Defining idea...

'**With your heads full of brains and your shoes full of feet,**
you're too smart to go down, any not-so-good street.
...Out there things can happen
and frequently do
to people as brainy
and footsy as you.'
DR SEUSS

How did it go?

Q You're kidding. I can't for the life of me touch my toes down in order. Does that mean I'm a freak?

A No, if you haven't worked your toes (even wiggling them works wonders) for a while, then they may not want to obey orders. You might find it helps to focus on the muscles to move if you touch the toes that aren't getting the message.

Q Ow. I get a cramp in the sole of my foot if I point and flex, what can I do about that?

A As you get used to more mobility in the foot that will go away. Try starting with your foot flat on the floor then very gently arching it with the toes and heel still touching the floor. That may provoke cramp in which case stop but if you do it progressively it will ease the cramp and may make you less likely to cramp in other foot flexing activities – like swimming.

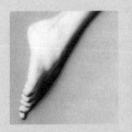 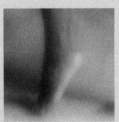 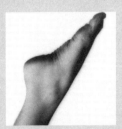

14

Playing footsie

There's more to practising your footsie than fine-tuning your under-table flirting.

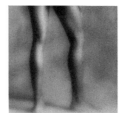

Your feet are marvels of biomechanics and in order to keep them that way you need to start working at the muscles that control foot flexion and extension — or in other words that point your toes up or down.

It's hard to tell from looking at it, but some of the key muscles that point and flex your foot are found in the shin. Not only are these muscles all but invisible, they're also notoriously hard to single out for exercise and most of us just don't bother. After all, if you're using your foot you're using your ankle and therefore the muscles of the shin. Except that sometimes the simple fact of walking around isn't enough to keep those muscles in trim and injury occurs. All of the following exercises are actually taken from rehabilitation programmes designed for runners. It's a fair bet that if you show me a runner who knows what his or her peroneus is, then I'll show you a runner who's suffered from shin splints. It's a debilitating injury caused by shock to the muscles of the shin and their attachments to the bone underneath. It's also quite difficult to work with because the shin doesn't exactly lend itself to stretching. Which is where these exercises come in.

By playing footsie you can exercise your ankle and shins anytime and anywhere. Obviously footsie is a lot more fun if you're across the table from someone you find significantly attractive. Except that back in the real world if I relied on romantic moments for my workouts I'd have wasted away by now. Here's an alternative.

Kick your shoes off and slowly write the entire alphabet, letter by letter, with your toes on the floor. Drawing every letter will have you bending your foot pretty much every which way. Of course if you happen to be an Arabic or Mandarin writer, then you're going to end up with shins like Stallone's biceps. When you've finished don't forget to repeat the sequence with the other foot. As well as exercising your shin muscles, playing footsie is a great little stress buster and highly recommended if you're stuck behind a desk.

SHIN STRETCH

Stretching the shin is harder to do than you might think because while straightening your foot and pointing your toes will extend the shin, it doesn't put much of a stretch on. To stretch it, make sure you're wearing comfy trainers and start by standing with feet hip-width apart, knees slightly bent. Then take a step backwards with one leg but keep the weight on your front foot. Now with the back foot tuck your toes under so that instead of standing with the ball of the foot on the ground, the tops of your toes are touching the ground. Very lightly bend your knees, lowering your body and pushing those toes into the ground to stretch the shin.

FOOT WEIGHTS

You might not think it possible to do weights with your foot but it is, although it takes a bit of ingenuity. Don't think about ankle weights since they will mainly affect the muscles that operate the knee. There are ways, however. Even a paint tin can be used for foot strength if it's the type that has a handle. Simply point your foot and put it through the loop of the handle and lift your leg so the paint tin is hanging from the pointed foot. Now lift the tin by flexing the foot and you may actually feel the shin muscles (see, believe me now?).

For more on ways of working the smaller muscles of the legs with resistance bands, try turning to IDEA 32, *Your flexible friend II.*

Try another idea...

RESISTANCE ISN'T FUTILE

The best way of exercising your feet is with resistance bands (see IDEA 32, *Your flexible friend II*). They're cheap, they're easy to pack away when you're on the move, they're fun to play with, and if it wasn't for the fact that they're quite hard to explain to customs officers when you get stopped they would be just about perfect. For foot muscles they're pretty much the only choice.

Wrap a resistance band around the ball of your foot with the ends in your hand, like reins. Now you can stretch the foot and work the muscles in every direction by pointing it down and away from you, pointing the toes, or turning the ankles outwards and inwards in either direction.

Having suffered shin splints myself I can vouch for the usefulness of this exercise in getting you back on your feet. Along with anyone else who's ever suffered shin splints, be they dancers, runners or football players, I can also assure you that if you've ever been there you will be prepared to spend a fair amount of time doing daft little things like this in order to help make sure you never go back there again.

'Heaven is under our feet as well as over our heads.'
HENRY DAVID THOREAU

Defining idea...

Q **Loved it but I find that writing out the whole alphabet with my toes is a tad time consuming. Can't you suggest something quicker that I can do when I just have a second?**

A *If you have only a couple of seconds free here or there during the day just try writing the word 'zoom'. Try it and you'll understand why.*

Q **You're not wrong, I'm only reading this because I have niggles in my shin. Should I still do the above?**

A *If you think you're on your way to shin splints you should see a sports doctor. If you keep hammering at them it can lead to stress fractures of the bone. That said, you'll know if you've got that far. In most cases, however, if you have light niggles in the muscles of the shin try icing the leg (ah, the wonder of a bag of frozen peas) and trying the alphabet writing – it's impact free and low intensity and can work wonders.*

15

Drop and give me twenty...oh all right, three

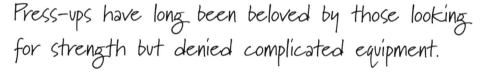

Press-ups probably remind you more of tattoos, drill sergeants and the good old days back in D Wing rather than the refined atmosphere of the Pilates studio. Nonetheless the press-up is a Pilates exercise – with a twist of course.

Press-ups have long been beloved by those looking for strength but denied complicated equipment.

Of course many such people are also denied access to belts, shoelaces and sharp instruments but it shouldn't come as too much of a surprise to see the press-up included in Joseph H. Pilates' first book of floor exercises, *Return to Life Through Contrology*.

The press-up lends itself perfectly to the Pilates ethos. It works a number of muscles simultaneously, notably the pectorals of the chest and the deltoids of the shoulder, but also the triceps at the back of the arm. Done correctly it encourages good Pilates posture, with a strong back and scooped stomach. There are a couple of points about the Pilates push-up, however, that would have them staring at you in

Here's an idea for you... **Take this technique further by doing the same move but instead of having your arms in line with each other and the shoulders, try moving one hand forwards and the other back. It's very important to maintain a straight spine and neutral pelvis for this because it puts the body slightly off balance and creates a slight twisting motion. What that's good for, however, is that it makes your arm muscles work in a different way, and brings in the oblique muscles to work on counteracting the twist.**

the punishment block. The first is that while no self-respecting hard man would admit to doing fewer than 50 press-ups at a go, Joseph H. recommends you repeat the exercise just three times. As ever, the emphasis in Pilates is on good form, smooth fluid motion and breathing, rather than simply forcing the muscles to repeat over and over to exhaustion. The other is that the full Pilates press-up starts standing up and bent over, walking the arms out to reach the normal press-up position. That too is typically Joseph, choosing to combine a back and hamstring stretch with the exercise, very much in line with his admiration of cats and the way that they stretch before embarking on movement.

The full Pilates press-up goes as follows.

Standing in neutral with feet together, bend over smoothly and try to touch the floor; if you can put your palms flat on the floor so much the better. 'Walk' your hands out away from you forwards, until you are stretched out in the classic press-up position with your arms shoulder-width apart and your hands pointed straight out forwards. Your weight should be on the toes and hands. Your body should be rigid and form a straight line from head to heels with your stomach scooped (see IDEA 5, *Scoop!*) and your pelvis in neutral (see IDEA 6, *Parking in neutral*). The neck should extend out forwards as far as possible. Now inhale slowly and lower the

body, keeping the back rigid, until your chin meets the floor. Then exhale slowly as you smoothly lift the body back to the start position by extending the arms.
Repeat three times.

While anyone with tattoos will sniff at the thought of doing a mere three press-ups, the fact is that for a lot of us even a single full-length press-up is either impossible, or impossible to do with the fluid control required for a Pilates move. If that sounds familiar, then make it easier on yourself by performing the move as a 'box press-up' in which you rest your knees on the ground to make it easier to bear the weight. If you do that, then you will have to be very careful about form and at first you will need either an instructor, a well-informed observer or a mirror because a lot of us when on our knees tend to drop our lower backs and/or stick our bums up in the air. Leaving aside the aesthetics of the position, the fact is that it leaves the pelvis hopelessly tilted and so puts a lot more strain on the spine.

If you like the idea of toned chest and triceps but don't feel strong enough for the full Pilates press-up, then take a look at press-ups using the Swiss ball in IDEA 30?

Try another idea...

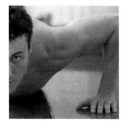

'Be sure never to repeat the selected exercise(s) more than the prescribed number of times since more harm will result than good by your unwittingly or intentionally disregarding this most important advice and direction.'
JOSEPH H. PILATES, laying down the law for those who would normally expect to pump out 50 or more press-ups.

Defining idea...

How did it go?

Q I can do press-ups till the cows come home but I can't for the life of me bend down and touch the floor, or even my own shins. Can I skip that bit?

A   *If you don't have the flexibility to do that part of the movement, then it's better to leave it out and work on back flexibility and stretches. If, as it sounds, you are a strong individual and yet you don't have the flexibility to bend and touch the floor, then you may also have built up imbalances in your body by overtraining some muscles at the expense of others. See a qualified Pilates practitioner for more advice.*

Q I find the box press-up too easy, and yet the full press-up too hard to do with the control required. Is there a halfway house?

A   *Yes, if you use a Swiss ball (see IDEA 30, On the ball II) because you can have the ball anywhere from your thighs down to your ankles which gives you a sliding scale of difficulty.*

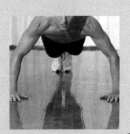

16

Getting smart with dumbbells I: Curly wurly

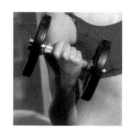

You probably thought dumbbells were named for the people who use them. With more and more instructors bringing weights into the studio here's the low-down on pumpin' iron the Pilates way.

Pilates purists look away now. Joseph H. never personally advocated the use of dumbbells for his exercises, and for those whose image of Pilates is all leotards and nary a drop of sweat in sight, then what follows is heresy and in all probability profoundly distasteful.

The fact is that while the Pilates purists have every right and reason to stick to the original set of exercises, the life force of Pilates has been such that it has evolved and expanded in ways that its founder may never have imagined. Whatever he would have made of it himself, his legacy goes far beyond the exercises he laid down. Exercise enthusiasts from all sorts of backgrounds have picked up on the principles behind Pilates and run with them. Literally in some cases. It was

Here's an idea for you... **One tip from the bodybuilders that doesn't clash with the Pilates approach is to vary the exercises from time to time so that you surprise your muscles into working differently. Wrapping a sweat towel around the bar so that it becomes thick (and soft) is one way of doing that because it changes your grip which may make you realise how even in an 'isolation' exercise like the curl you are still using other muscles, in this case in the forearm.**

inevitable that even pumpin' iron would get a touch of the Pilates brush, and weights are fast making their way into the studios. Anyone who does or has used weights has a lot to learn from applying Pilates principles to their pump. And anyone who is used to classical Pilates mat work will find that weights, used intelligently, can add the resistance that Joseph sought by using his elaborate machines. With the difference that few of us can afford to have a Pilates machine in the house, let alone tuck it under the bed when it's not wanted and maintain it with a lick of paint every half century.

There are eight principals of Pilates, and number seven is 'isolation' – the ability to single out one muscle at a time and work it and it alone. This is something that even the most muscle-bound meathead in the gym can understand because while compound exercises (involving several muscles) build power, isolating an individual muscle ('targeting' it in bodybuilding parlance) is the way to work it to exhaustion and build it. Dumbbells are excellent for that. The difference is that in Pilates the aim is never to pump up a muscle but instead to lengthen and strengthen it. In practice that means that the bodybuilder and the Pilates practitioner may make almost the same movement, but where the bodybuilder aims for the biggest weight they can lift, the Pilates goal is the best possible form using light weights and few repetitions.

CURLY WURLY

The basic bicep isolation exercise is the curl. It comes in many variations but the bottom line is that you bend the elbow so the fist rises up to meet the shoulder. Here we'll consider two ways of curling: standing, which is what you'll do in a class, and sitting, which is what you may choose to do in the gym or at home.

Standing curls are very simple as long as you remember basic Pilates form. Your feet should be hip-width apart, your knees very slightly bent (never locked) and your pelvis in neutral (of course you know that by now, but I will be drummed out of Pilates world if I fail to mention it). Your shoulders should be relaxed but not slumped and you should have a light dumbbell in each hand. Don't forget to scoop that stomach (see IDEA 5, *Scoop!*).

Women are very good at selecting a light dumbbell. Blokes still feel that ancestral call of the caveman and try to reach for the biggest ones they think they'll get away with. Here's some advice. If you're in a class, then look around for the hardest looking woman you can see. Yes her, with the Hell's Angels tattoos. See what weight she's holding? Good. Now look for the nearest woman old enough to be her mum. You should be holding whatever Hell's Grandma is using.

You don't have a minute to lose. Now you've worked your biceps you simply have to turn to IDEA 17, *Getting smart with dumbbells II*, and work the back of your arm or else you'll end up all unbalanced and out of whack.

Try another idea...

'*The last three or four reps is what makes the muscle grow. This area of pain divides the champion from someone else who is not a champion.*'
ARNOLD SCHWARZENEGGER, not a man pursuing the long, lean look

Defining idea...

The lift starts with the weight at your sides, your palms facing inwards toward your thighs. Start to exhale and lift one arm at a time in a smooth, controlled way. The elbow bends and the hand and weight lift up in what's called a hammer grip (the bar of the weight vertical in the fist), then, as your elbow reaches 90 degrees and your forearm is parallel with the floor, you slowly turn your wrist as you continue to lift so that at the top of the movement your palm finishes turned in towards your shoulder. The whole lift is done in one long exhale. At the top start to inhale slowly and let the arm go back down the same way, reversing the wrist twist so that you end up again with your palm facing your thigh. The down movement should take just as long as the up movement. Now perform the same action with the other hand. Five repetitions of each is all you're going to do.

The sitting version of the curl is the same but some people feel more comfortable with it, and if that means you can concentrate more on what your biceps are doing, then so much the better. Sit with your pelvis in neutral and your feet flat on the floor. Scoop, and then follow the exercise instructions as above for five repetitions of each arm.

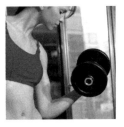 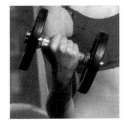

Q **I think I'm isolating the biceps but I can feel exercise in my shoulders. That can't be right can it?**

A *Watch yourself in a mirror as you perform the curls. My bet is that you're not keeping your arms straight by your sides and as you curl upwards you're allowing your elbow to come out sideways which brings the deltoid muscle of the shoulder into play. It's a great muscle, but it's not needed now so keep your elbows tucked in.*

Q **I've heard that you should vary dumbbell exercises to get better results. Is that true? And if so, how do I vary this one?**

A *Yes it's true. Your muscles quickly adapt to resistance work so it's very much part of the Pilates philosophy to change your routine and make them 'think' a bit. For a variant try performing the whole curl with the hammer grip so your palms never turn inwards towards your shoulders.*

How did it go?

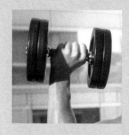 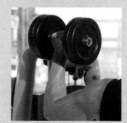

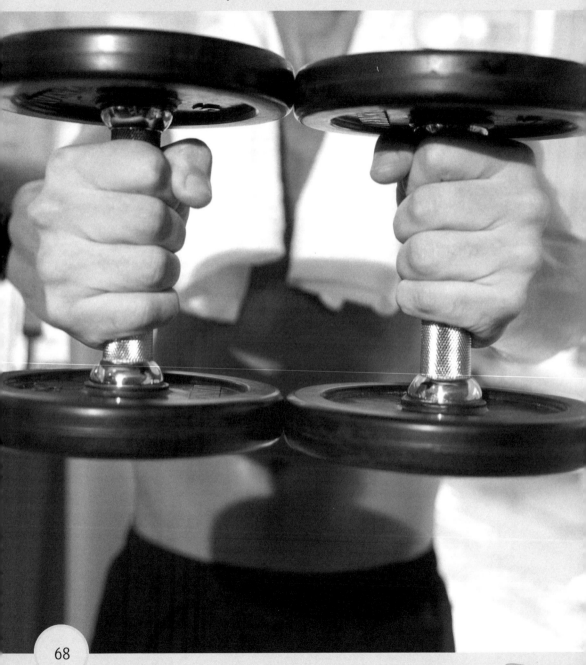

17

Getting smart with dumbbells II: Tri harder

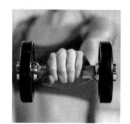

It takes two to tango. Although isolation is a great technique for working individual muscles you have to remember to do the same with their partners or they'll sulk and you'll end up all out of whack.

In Idea 16, 'Getting smart with dumbbells I', we looked at the biceps. The biceps run down the front of your upper arm, but you know that already from Popeye.

Now it's time to look at the triceps, which run down the back of your upper arm. Although we'll be doing separate exercises designed to target one muscle at a time, it's best to work the two together because they complement each other – the biceps bends the arm at the elbow, the triceps straightens it.

The basic rules of weight lifting with Pilates remain exactly as before. The spine is always neutral. The stomach is always scooped to engage the transversus and lower abdominals, and the weights are light because this is not about working to fatigue.

Here's an idea for you...

As well as strengthening your muscles with weights it's always a good idea to stretch them. Providing your muscles are 'warm', as they should be after a weight work out, you can go into a type of stretch called a developmental stretch which aims to lengthen the muscle. For the triceps this starts off just as the previous exercise only without the weight. Put your right arm straight up in the air, then bend at the elbow so your hand is behind your neck. Now with the left arm reach across, take the bent elbow in your hand and gently pull in the direction of the left shoulder. As you feel the stretch come in, hold it there for a count of eight seconds and feel the muscle relax into that stretch. Then gently pull a bit deeper into the stretch and count for a further 12–20 seconds in order to extend the muscles further.

Joseph H. actually believed that working to fatigue released poisons into the muscle and while that might sound daft it's worth bearing in mind that the point at which muscles 'fail' due to fatigue is down to the build up of lactic acid. The Pilates belief is that it is never necessary to exhaust a muscle for the sake of developing it and so even when working with dumbbells the rule is to focus on taking a muscle through its movement as completely, and fluidly, as possible. Neither heavy weights nor high repetitions figure in this philosophy. Equally it is a point of Pilates practice that the lift and the descent with a weight should take the same time, exhaling through the effort, and inhaling with the return.

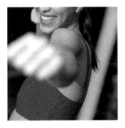

TIME TO TRY THE TRICEPS

Stand in neutral, feet hip-width apart, knees slightly bent, shoulders relaxed but not slumped, and scoop your stomach for core strength. With a light weight (gentlemen in particular kindly observe the note on weights in IDEA 16, *Getting smart with dumbbells I*) in one hand only, put that arm straight up in the air and now smoothly bend the elbow so the dumbbell comes to rest behind your head at the back of your neck. Exhale and smoothly straighten your arm. The upper arm should remain completely motionless with the only movement coming from the elbow. Keep your shoulder out straight so as to ensure the chest and airways are opened up, and make sure the wrist is straight and doesn't twist or bend at all during the movement. When you get to the top of the movement your arm and the weight should be straight up in the air again. Don't lock the elbow at the top of the move. Inhale as you bring the weight back down again to behind the neck. Each completed raise is a repetition. After five repetitions switch hands and repeat for the other side (this is all about balance so it's important to work both arms equally).

Looking to improve strength and resistance to injury in your forearms? Then go to IDEA 48, *Forearm smash*, to learn more.

Try another idea...

'Inward calm cannot be maintained unless physical strength is constantly and intelligently replenished.'
Buddhist words of wisdom

Defining idea...

How did it go?

Q   How do I avoid feeling cramped and constricted between my shoulder and my neck as I perform the exercise?

A   *You're tensing your trapezius muscle. Take the arm further away from the neck by straightening your shoulders. Right at the start, when you put your arm straight up in the air, you have probably shrugged your shoulders upwards. Stop at that point, look at yourself in a mirror, and without moving the arm at all try to lower the shoulder so it's back in line with the non-lifting shoulder. Think about sliding your shoulder blades down and outwards before you start to lift as this will reduce the stress. Finally extend the neck as if you were being pulled up by a string running right through your spine and out the top of your head.*

Q   Should I feel tiredness in my wrist after the exercise?

A   *No, it sounds as if you may have let your wrist go loose during the exercise instead of keeping it firm and straight. It's a common problem among those who are used to using heavier weights as the light weights of Pilates are so 'easy' that your concentration may wander, leading to poor form. Remember that the essence of the move is not working hard but working smart, so concentrate absolutely on your form.*

18

Man and machine

Machines have always played a part in Pilates. Joseph Pilates developed many of his techniques using makeshift machines made out of mattresses and bedsprings.

Pilates' own ideas on the perfect resistance machines would later take shape in the form of the Reformer and the Cadillac (see Ideas 36 and 39) but I suspect he would have approved of the weights machines found in pretty much every gym.

Free weights (dumbbells and barbells) have the distinct advantage of a greater range of movement and the recruitment of stabilising and balancing muscles to do the work. But you have to know what you're doing or you risk injury. Plus the testosterone-charged atmosphere of most free weight rooms is seriously off-putting. Machine weights, on the other hand, are designed to make it as difficult as possible to complete the exercise badly. They make it nigh on impossible to drop weights on yourself (or others), they often have instructions and illustrations, and they are much less intimidating to use.

Here's an idea for you...

Cable stations are an excellent way of working, similar in concept to Joseph Pilates' Pedipull machine in that they provide constant tension. Think for a moment of a barbell curl (see IDEA 16, *Getting smart with dumbbells I*). The weight is heavy as you bend your arm upwards but as soon as it reaches vertical your bicep stops working and the lift is finished. Now imagine doing the same curl but with a cable lifting a weight via a pulley. Even when you reach the top of the lift, the pulley and weight means the cable is trying to pull back out of your hands. That's constant resistance and a great way to work. Remembering your Pilates positioning (feet flat, knees relaxed, neutral and scoop), try curls with a low pulley (cable rises from the ground) or triceps push-downs from a high pulley. For the latter, start standing a step away from the machine with your elbows at right angles, forearms parallel to the floor. The bar should be pulling upwards in your hands. Now exhale and push it down using only your forearms bending at the elbow. Inhale and bring it back to the start position to finish.

The illustration here is of a bench press machine, but the essential Pilates approach is as true whether the machine in question is a shoulder press, a pec deck or a seated chest press.

The bench press primarily works the muscles of the chest and the deltoids at the front of your shoulders, but because it's a pushing exercise it also recruits the triceps. What people often forget is that the back muscles are also part of this – they provide a solid 'launch pad' to push from – which is another reason why perfect form makes all the difference. Even powerlifters agree that getting technique right is the key to building strength.

First of all make absolutely sure that the machine is set up correctly for you. That's not just a matter of getting the weight right – it's also about adjusting seats, seat backs and benches until you feel comfortable with the positioning of handles. In the case of the bench press you should lie down with your feet flat on the floor. Your spine should be in neutral and your shoulders relaxed so you can feel the bench with the middle of the back between the shoulder blades. Take a grip on the handles (don't try and lift anything yet) and look at the angle of your arms at the elbow. If it's around 90 degrees that's fine, but if your elbows are dipped down below the level of your shoulders, then don't attempt to lift the weight. See if you can lower the height of the bench, or change the position of the handles. If you lift the weight from a position where your elbows are back behind your shoulders you risk putting extreme stress on the chest and shoulder muscles and will almost certainly stress your back in the effort. Now get up again and go to the weight stack. Slot the pin into the correct hole to choose a comfortable weight, remembering that this is about form, not about bench pressing your own bodyweight. If you don't know what is likely to be comfortable, then aim low – it's much easier to go back and increase a weight than it is recover from the strain of trying to lift something too heavy.

Go back to the bench and lie down. Scoop your stomach, check again that your feet are flat on the floor and exhale as you push the bar away from you, straightening the arms but stopping the movement without locking your elbows.

If you're interested in resistance machines and have access to a well-equipped Pilates studio, then it may be time to try the machines designed by Joseph Pilates himself. Take a look at IDEA 36, *Rack and roll with the Reformer*.

Try another idea...

'The resistance that you fight physically in the gym and the resistance that you fight in life can only build a strong character.'
ARNOLD SCHWARZENEGGER

Defining idea...

Make sure your wrists are straight and firm throughout. Watch out for any arching of the spine – there should be none. Inhale as you bring the bar back down and stop before the weight you lifted crashes back down on the weight stack. If your sole aim is Pilates technique, then three to five repetitions will be fine. If you're looking to incorporate Pilates form into your normal weightlifting, then be very careful as you increase weights because the temptation will be to forget about form in the struggle to lift heavier weights.

**Pilates meets
pumping iron.**
*A little more toning, a
little less testosterone.*

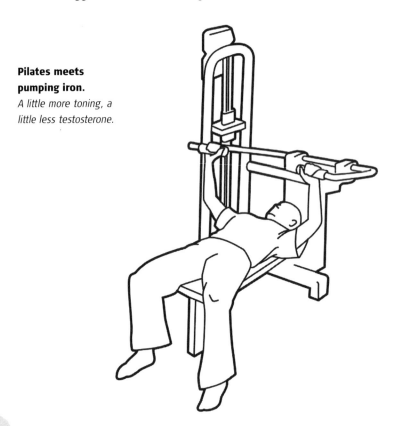

Q **I get a red mark and even bloodspots on my shoulder blades. What's up?**

How did it go?

A *It means you're lifting a very heavy weight and not using the full platform of your back to do so. Leaving aside the wisdom of the weight itself, try and look in a mirror next time you bench press. As you push to get to the top of the lift you are probably pushing down with your shoulder blades rather than your whole back. As this pushes the ribcage up, the small of your back will part contact with the bench which makes your core weaker and more liable to injury.*

Q **I see other people lifting their feet up and putting them on the bench. Is this right?**

A *Not really. There is a belief that it works the core more but for a weight exercise stability is the key to success and putting your feet on the bench doesn't help. Nor for that matter does tapping them, or letting them dance around, both of which you will sometimes see people do.*

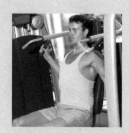

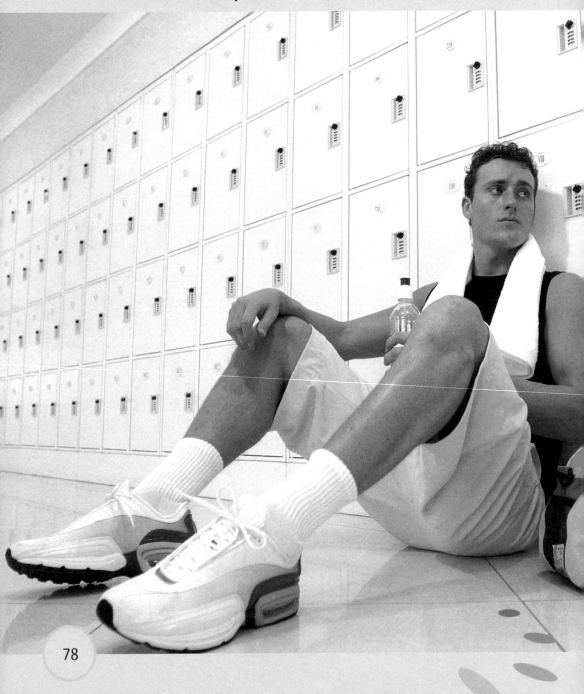

19

Are we nearly there yet?

Let me guess: you really enjoyed Pilates when you first tried it but now you've lost your way a little and have stopped taking classes or practising at home. Sound familiar? Then you need some goals.

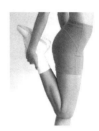

There's a moment in 'Sex and the City' when Samantha's naked rear end provokes an admiring gasp. She smiles and mouths the single word, 'Pilates'.

I don't have any statistics but I'll take a wild guess that the number of people showing up to Pilates classes skyrocketed that week. The original clients for Joseph H.'s techniques were dancers looking to shake off injuries. Rehabilitation is still one of the big reasons for going and for those people the goal is simple – you do it until you get better. These days, however, people turn to Pilates for all sorts of reasons ranging from the quest for better self-knowledge, to the search for a different kind of musculature and mobility, and probably more often than not the promises of a toned tum and lean legs. All of which are perfectly admirable but if you want to get to a goal you'd best be sure just where it is you think you're going.

One of the biggest problems for most of us coming to Pilates is being sure that we're getting what we want out of it. Proper Pilates instruction is expensive (for good reason – see IDEA 2, *Picking your Pilates instructor*) and there is the potential problem that while everyone I know who tried it raves about the feeling of

Here's an idea for you...

Ever thought of blackmail? Well now's the time. There's a website called 'Hot or Not?' (www.hotornot.com) where people post pictures of themselves and invite the world to comment on whether they're hot. Or not.

So what's that got to do with you? Simple. Take that digital image of yourself from the above, give it to a friend, along with the permission for them to post it on 'Hot or Not' if you don't supply one of you looking better in time for your self-appointed deadline. As well as posting that picture, they should also email the people you know and invite them to go to the site and comment. Motivation enough to do something?

calmness and being energised, there are also large numbers of people who try it, like it and yet drift away. Part of that is the problem that if you don't know what you're looking for, then you won't recognise it when you get there. The answer? Set out your goals so you can congratulate yourself as you go along. Do the following tests, set yourself a deadline (three months from now? six months?) and compare the before and the after.

LOSING WEIGHT

First off don't think about losing weight – it's a sham. Muscle is denser than fat so if you replace fat with lovely lean muscle you'll actually weigh more. Bin the scales and instead find out your body composition either from a gym or your doctor, or by using a fat monitor. Instead of weight, aim to lose a target percentage of fat by a set date.

SHAPING UP

This is one of the trickiest of the lot because when we look in the mirror we filter what we see through how we feel. Feeling good? Then you'll probably find you look better. Since Pilates undoubtedly makes people feel more relaxed and energised it's no wonder they think they look better. To be sure, though, you'll need some way of checking how you look now, with how you looked then.

You'll find more on how to stretch yourself in IDEA 40, Roll out the barrel.

Try another idea...

In this day of digital cameras we can all take instant pictures that come with dates attached. If you don't have a digital camera an ordinary one will do but make a note of the date. Now you may need an assistant as you will want to strip to your underwear and have a picture taken of your body, or your selected body part, in order to see if you are having any effect. You may be able to manage this solo with the aid of a mirror. The important thing here is to make a note of the place and the lighting so you can reproduce exactly the same lighting again later. Indirect lighting from above will make you look more ripped and rippled with lean muscle because it throws shadows that highlight the sinews. That's fine but don't make the mistake of having sympathetic lighting in your 'before' shot and harsh lighting in the 'after'.

'After 10 sessions you'll feel a difference, after 20 sessions you'll see a difference, and after 30 sessions everyone will see a difference.'
JOSEPH H. PILATES

Defining idea...

HEIGHT

People often say that Pilates makes them feel taller. Much of this is down to a shift in posture, so that you stand taller. Why not measure yourself against the wall with a pencil mark? To make it accurate you should get someone else to do it and you should stand as you normally do, not strain upwards. Likewise for the 'after' measurement. Remember to take the measurement at the same time of day – just after getting out of bed – because we can shrink by a centimetre during a day on our feet.

How did it go?

Q   I tried the fat monitor and don't seem to have lost any. Can I give up now?

A   *No! Firstly, don't forget all the other reasons you do this – the self-respect, the good feeling, etc. Secondly, remember that fat monitors do give different figures depending on the time of day, the amount of water you've drunk and the point of your menstrual cycle. Are you sure you're comparing like with like?*

Q   My instructor keeps stressing flexibility as a goal. I have no urge to do the splits so is this really a waste of time? How will I know if I'm making progress anyway?

A   *Over time collagen forms links in the tissues of the muscles and reduces flexibility. This limits our range of movement and greatly speeds up ageing but it can be turned back and Pilates is excellent for that. Most people feel benefits within only a couple of months of regular sessions.*

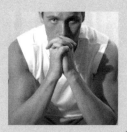

20

Hundreds and thousands

The Hundred is one of the basic mat work moves, but with a sprinkling of variations it quickly becomes a range of killer workouts for the abdominals. Tum toning time.

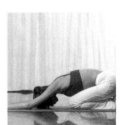

The Hundred is the very first exercise featured in Joseph Pilate's 'Return to Life through Contrology' and has been a mainstay of mat work ever since.

Arguably the classic Pilates abdominal exercise, it has been picked up and played with by generations of Pilates practitioners with the result that there are now a whole host of options to make it harder, easier or more concerned with co-ordination. Of course what they really needed to do was to change its name because there is nothing more guaranteed to make the heart sink than the idea of doing a hundred of anything. Until some bright spark comes up with a more laid-back label, here's a handful of Hundreds for you to pick from and play with until you're sore or have abs like a cattle grid, whichever comes first.

THE STANDARD

This one you should already know but I'm including it as the reference so you can understand how the others differ.

Here's an idea for you...

As well as being an abs exercise *par excellence* the Hundred is a serious breathing exercise since the idea is to breathe wide into the back rather than have the chest or abdomen rise and fall. One little trick you can try to work on both wide breathing and scooping the stomach is to balance a tennis ball on your lower belly in between your belly button and the naughty bits. To keep it there without it moving you'll need to focus on breathing laterally so the sides of your ribcage go in and out rather than the front rising and falling. It will also remind you to keep your lower abs locked down even as you work them.

Lie flat on the floor and raise your legs straight up in the air. If that's already too tough or your hamstrings are too tight to be comfortable with your legs straight up, then bend your knees 90 degrees so your lower legs are now parallel with the ground. At this point you should look like someone who's overdone it at a dinner party, tipped their chair over backwards and is now staring at the ceiling, trying to work out where all the other guests have gone.

Make sure your pelvis is in neutral, your stomach scooped. Your arms should be straight down at your sides, palms downwards. Curl your head up so your shoulders are off the ground and you are looking down your body. Think of that dinner party guest finally working out where everyone else is. Don't drop your chin into your chest, instead imagine you have an apple between your chin and your chest and don't squash it or let it roll off. Breathing in and breathing wide, pump your arms up and down about 15 cm (6 inches) off the floor. Keep your arms straight from shoulder to fingertip. Breath out and repeat the action another five times. Breath in for another five. Keep count of those stiff-arm air-slaps and when you hit a hundred you can curl your head back down and relax. I recommend a good stretch with your arms as far above your head as you can get while making the body as long as possible. 'Never exceed a hundred movements' was Joseph's original recommendation, just in case you were getting a bit carried away there.

Joseph's Hundred too easy for you? If you have abs of iron, then IDEA 21, *The Hundred – doing the ton (part two)*, is calling out to you to come and have a go – if you think you're hard enough.

Try another idea...

THE ORIGINAL

Joseph Pilates' original Hundred suggested starting out with only 20 repetitions. There again, one key difference between his technique and the one we normally see today is that he had the arms out at nearly 45 degrees, and most importantly had both legs out straight but lifted 5 cm (2 inches) off the ground throughout the whole exercise. Try it. Feel the difference? Having the legs straight and slightly off the ground really ups the ante on the abs. This position is often considered too tough for beginners, and it makes keeping the pelvis in neutral both hard work and essential to avoid straining the back.

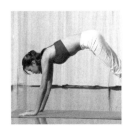

'I think and think for months and years. Ninety-nine times, the conclusion is false. The hundredth time I am right.'
ALBERT EINSTEIN

Defining idea...

How did it go?

Q   In our class we don't lift the head off the ground. I tried it but find it very hard. Is there an easier way?

A   *Certainly, if your neck isn't strong enough (yet) to support the head without stress, then try to lift up for the exhaled five pulses, and rest it back on the mat for the inhaled five.*

Q   I'm keeping my knees bent but having trouble keeping my back flat, am I doing something wrong?

A   *Check the position of your feet. Without realising it you've probably angled your thighs so that your knee isn't at right angles any more – either bringing the knees into your chest or letting the knees drop down slightly. The first will tip your pelvis forward, the latter tips it back. Either way you'll be out of neutral and your spine will arch.*

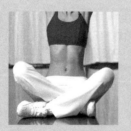
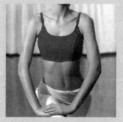

21

The Hundred – doing the ton (part two)

Joseph's original Hundred too easy for you? Well bring it on then, here's the Hundred for the hard core.

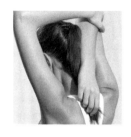

More Hundreds? Well yes, that's the thing about Hundreds, they just go on and on. Just when you think you've got the thing cracked, another one comes along.

The fact that there are ever harder variations on the Hundred tells us a fair amount about the innate perversity of the human psyche, but most of all it speaks volumes about what people are prepared to put themselves through in the search for a svelte stomach.

Once you've mastered the traditional Hundred, and Joseph's original version with the legs just off the ground (see IDEA 20, *Hundreds and Thousands*), there are a number of movements you can add to make you focus more on the co-ordination of different parts of the body and to make that mind-to-muscle connection so crucial for individual muscle control.

Here's an idea for you...

Get hip. As well as thighs, shoulders and abs, the Hundred can also be adapted to include hip mobility while working the waistline. This variation takes both concentration and strong muscles to get right, which means keeping it smooth and controlled. If you rush it you'll end up losing your neutral position. Plus the fact that with your legs twitching away in the air you'll look like a dying housefly.

Start as before flat on your back and raise both legs in the air. Scoop the stomach, park the pelvis, exhale and curl the head up. This time the leg movement is circular. Keeping the legs straight (but trying not to lock out the knee), scissor them (one goes forward, one back) and with the right leg describe a semicircle going down so your leg ends up at 45 degrees from the floor while the left leg makes a semicircle going up towards your face. That's one repetition (and therefore a five-second count with hand air-slaps) before reversing the position to swap the legs. The trick is that despite the fact that the legs are swivelling at the hip, your hips should not tilt – which gives your abs one more thing to worry about.

The standard Hundred concentrates on holding the abs in tight and only moving the arms from the shoulders. These variations add to the fun by bringing in leg movements. This not only adds to the workload of the stomach muscles, but also the adductor and abductor muscles of the inner thighs. In addition, if the legs are moved alternately rather than together it also works the oblique muscles that run down the sides of the stomach.

ALTERNATING LEGS

Start off on the floor in the usual position. Pelvis in neutral, neck long, arms straight down by your sides. Now bring the legs in to the chest, keeping your back down on the floor as you do so. Scoop your stomach and straighten both legs so they're pointing straight up in the air, the feet pointed but not overstretched so that your toes are curled up in a claw. Check that your pelvis is still parked in neutral. Now exhale and curl your head up (see IDEA 20, *Hundreds and thousands*). At the same time lower one leg only down towards the floor. Only go as far down as you can without your back arching. The movement should be completely smooth, not jerky or bouncy, and you should be able to pump the arms as with the traditional Hundred five times with each leg lower. Breath in as you raise the raise the leg back to the upright position, pumping the hands again for five, then swap legs and repeat. Keep the shoulder blades off the ground for the duration of the exercise.

Enjoy the hip mobility and control? Then maybe you should try IDEA 22, *Take that!*

Try another idea...

V LEGS

This is like a conventional Hundred, but where normally you would keep your legs out straight and together, here you open them to form a V for a count of five seconds as you 'mark time' with arms pumping up and down, and then close your legs. Moving the legs adds to the workload of the abs, and opening and closing brings in the abductor (opening) and adductor muscles (closing). Once again the head is kept curled up and the shoulder blades off the ground throughout the exercise.

LEG LIFTS

Here you alternate positions between the standard Hundred with your legs straight up in the air, and a second position where you lower both legs down to the position of Joseph's original Hundred (see IDEA 20, *Hundreds and thousands*). Remember the five-second breath, and five counted air-slaps in each position.

'A man thinks as well through his legs and arms as his brain.'
HFNRY DAVID THOREAU

Defining idea...

Q   **I can really feel the contraction in my abs but I do find, unusually for Pilates, that it hurts a bit. Is there any way of easing that without giving up on the intensity?**

A   *You may want to stretch out your stomach first to lengthen the rectus abdominis and prepare it for the hard work of the Hundred. Try some exercises on your stomach, arching your back to get the stretch – see IDEA 44,* Bending over backwards.

Q   **When I do the scissors leg movement I feel a tightness on the front of my thigh leading to my groin. What's that all about?**

A   *Sounds like your hip flexors are tight. Try warming up by lying on your back and hugging your knees to your chest to help stretch them.*

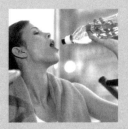 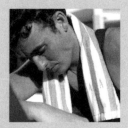

22

Take that!

Part ballet, part kickboxing, the kneeling side kick will open up your hips and fine-tune your balance. Just make sure the family cat is out of range before you let fly.

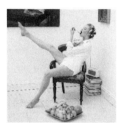

Although the vast majority of Pilates exercises are smooth and slow there is an exception to every rule and this is one of the few that Joseph H. specifically expected to be done quickly.

Because it's fast and forceful you're unlikely to come across it in most classes, and if your Pilates studio is a little on the compact and *bijou* side you're unlikely to come across it at all simply because of the free space required around each participant. It's a humdinger for the hips, great for getting your breathing going and works core strength because the swinging force is constantly threatening to unbalance you, meaning that all the muscles of the girdle of strength are working to maintain the pose. Just make sure that you're warmed up and well stretched before you give it a go because it requires a certain amount of flexibility. Try getting gung-ho with your groin muscles and you'll end up looking like you were on the receiving end of the kneeling side kick rather than the one dealing it out.

Here's an idea for you...

If you're happy with the normal kneeling side kick, then you can add to the imbalance slightly by taking your hand off your head and pointing it straight up into the air. Remember to focus on your spinal alignment – try to extend your neck in line with your spine. To increase the stretch on the obliques muscles of the side of your body, try bending the elbow slightly and letting the forearm drop so that it arcs over your head like a ballerina. A ballerina lying on the floor delivering vicious kicks like a drunken sailor perhaps, but a ballerina nonetheless.

Take up a kneeling position on the floor (as ever check your pelvic parking and your scoop), then stretch the right leg straight out sideways in line with the body and support your bodyweight with the left hand on the floor. Your toes should be pointed like a dancer, not curled over in a toe fist. Your arm should be quite straight but don't lock your elbow – keep it slightly flexed as it will absorb the movement better. Bend your right elbow and rest your right hand on your head.

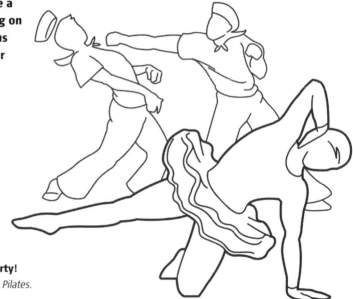

Sidekick – Take that and party!
Part ballet, part kickboxer, pure Pilates.

From that start position inhale quickly while swinging the right leg back, then exhale quickly and swing the leg forward again. Now switch sides and do the same with the left leg. Four forward and back swings with each leg completes the set.

The trick is not simply to unleash a scything side kick but to do so while maintaining the pelvis in position and resisting the rotational forces with the strength of your own abs. While it's easy to focus on the leg because it's obviously working, think of your body as being like a clock. The pendulum may be swinging to and fro, but the real artistry is in the subtle motion of the workings you can't see.

Before you start flinging limbs about in gay abandon you may want to learn a little more about your psoas muscle – take a look at IDEA 43, *So hip it hurts*, to learn more. If you're interested in strengthening you leg muscles, then as well as kicking movements you may want to look at weights – try IDEA 42, *Shake a leg*, to learn about leaner, longer, stronger limbs.

Try another idea...

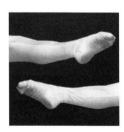

'As a general rule, do not kick the shins of the opposite gentleman under the table, if personally unacquainted with him.'
LEWIS CARROLL, on the delicate etiquette of letting fly with the low kick

Defining idea...

How did it go?

Q   I'm delivering a kick like a mule. But I feel like I'm permanently on the point of losing my balance. Am I overdoing it?

A   *That depends on how well you're controlling the imbalance but it does sound like you're pushing it a little. In his original instructions Joseph H. was explicit that this should be a dramatic movement. He instructed that you should swing each leg 'forcibly' and 'as far as possible' both on the back swing and the front swing. To the modern mind, however, a lot of his original instructions were a tad hardcore, especially for someone experimenting without the supervision of a qualified instructor. Remember that control is the key to every Pilates movement but the first time you try this you may want to take it a little easy. Slow the action down a little and concentrate on taking the leg through the full range of movement so that you're relying less on momentum and more on muscle.*

Q   I'm doing the advanced move with my arm forming an arc over my head but the resulting stretch isn't entirely comfortable. Any ideas?

A   *First off, any move that isn't comfortable means you should stop and think about what you're doing. Ideally you should do it under the supervision of an instructor to get them to spot faults in your technique. The most likely answer is that you're stretching the ribs but not extending the spine at the same time. Make sure you're trying to push your neck out in line with your spine, as if you were growing taller. For more on that see IDEA 37, A little bit on the side.*

23

Backs against the wall

Wall work provides a welcome break from the mat, a set of different sensations and can be done pretty much anywhere and anytime.

While you might reasonably have reservations about lying down on the floor in most places, you can practice your wall work pretty anywhere.

OK I guess if you live and work in an igloo or a tent then there are certain practical hurdles to overcome but in general the beauty of wall work is that if you can lean, you can learn.

We're an upright sort of beastie so it comes as no surprise that there's a very primitive, primeval sense of vulnerability about lying down. The word prone (which in exercise means lying face down) has strong connotations of being open to attack and most of us are very reluctant to get down on the floor to exercise if there's any chance of someone walking in. Even people we know well. Being upright, however, feels less exposed so I find I'm far more likely to make use of a spare five minutes with a little wall work than I am to sit or lie down to stretch.

You can combine the relaxing effects of rolling your spine off the wall with a strengthening exercise for your bum and the front of your thighs called **The Chair**. This is for when you've mastered rolling your spine and can concentrate on some strength work at the same time as unwinding. If you find the position interferes with the basic roll off the wall, then you should go back to the basic move until it is second nature. The move is exactly the same as rolling off the wall but your start position should be with the knees bent at right angles and the thighs parallel to the ground. Be careful that your knees don't project further forward than your feet, and that your bum doesn't drop below your knee level. From the side it should look as if you are sitting in an imaginary chair. Now complete your six repetitions of rolling your spine off the wall. The temptation will be to rush through the rolls, or cut corners because of the feeling of effort in your thighs. Try not to.

Not everyone's the same of course. There are always stories of businessmen setting down their suitcases in airport lounges and rolling like a ball (see IDEA 25, *Foetal attraction*).

Start off by standing 30 cm (12 inches) or more from a wall with your feet hip-width apart and your knees slightly bent. Now lean back into the wall so your bum touches it and press your back against the wall, extending the upper body from the hips upwards as if you wanted to grow taller (without straightening your legs). Feel for your leg muscles and make the effort to relax them. In particular try to relax the thigh muscles (quads), which tend to tense, and the hamstring at the back of your leg, which will be stretched by this move. Scoop the stomach, park the pelvis and relax the shoulders without slumping them. Try to slide the shoulder blades down your back rather than pulling them backwards as this way you'll feel the wall over much more of your back area. Scooping your stomach should also mean that you can feel the small of your back flatten against the wall. This is, however, a matter of personal physique and if your J-Lo style curves happen to prevent the small of your back from touching, then that's fine as long as your spine is in line.

Now breathe out and drop your chin to your chest. Start to peel yourself off the wall one vertebra at a time. Try to feel each one as it leaves the wall and you bend ever further forwards. Let your upper body hang forward and loose so your head is down towards your knees and your arms are hanging down towards the floor. Some people can touch the floor at this point, don't worry if you're not one of them – they may be particularly supple, or they may just have arms like gorillas. Just concentrate on releasing your own stress as you relax.

While simple wall work has that anytime, anywhere appeal, you can take it a step further with props in the studio or at home. Take a look at the wall exercise with the Swiss ball in IDEA 24, *Balls to the wall*, for more ideas on achieving backbone bliss while making friends with the masonry.

Try another idea...

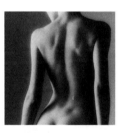

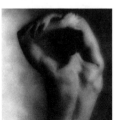

'A pat on the back, though only a few vertebrae removed from a kick in the pants, is miles ahead in results.'
ELLA WHEELER WILCOX, American critic

Defining idea...

97

The return move starts with the tailbone and the pelvis. Breathing in, think of dropping your tailbone and pulling the pelvis back to place the vertebrae of the lower spine back against the wall. Carry on placing each and every one back against the wall one at a time until you are where you started. Repeat six times.

Backs against the wall.
NB this is a Pilates pose, not a hold-up by the invisible man.

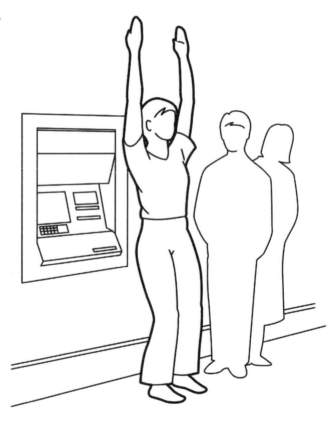

Q   Why don't my knees feel comfortable?

A   Check your foot position. When you bend your leg while exercising it's important not to let the knee project further forward than the foot. If it does so, the angle at the knee becomes more acute (smaller) than 90 degrees and this puts strain on the knee itself. It's very common for people to check their knee at what they think is the deepest point of a bend or stretch, and not notice that in fact they go beyond that point. The answer is simply to start with the foot placed further forward away from you.

Q   As I sit into The Chair I find my ankles want to leave the floor. Should I let them?

A   No, while this could be a sign of tight Achilles tendons you should try and keep the soles of your feet planted firmly on the floor (unless this causes pain of course). By doing so you make yourself more stable and stretch the Achilles which should help alleviate the problem in the future.

How did
it go?

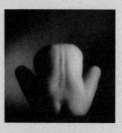 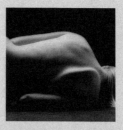

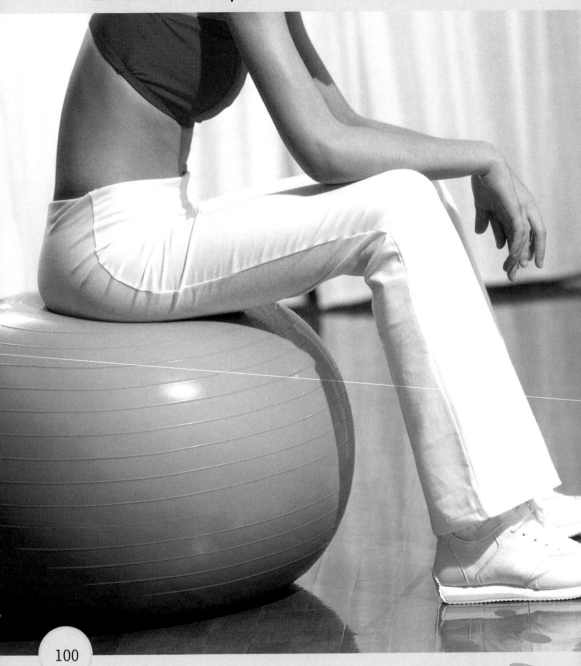

24

Balls to the wall

Take one ball plus one wall and you have a recipe for a superbly gentle way of working the muscles of the legs while keeping the spine in a state of bouncy backbone bliss.

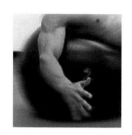

In Idea 23, 'Backs against the wall', you saw that walls can do so much more than stop the ceiling from falling on our heads. Here you'll look at how combining the wall with the Swiss ball can provide a workout for the thighs and bum while keeping the back beautifully supported.

Because the ball helps perform moves so much more smoothly this is also a great way for beginners to learn potentially tough moves, and for those feeling a little sore or stiff to gently ease those thigh muscles.

First find your wall. Since we're working with our globular friend the Swiss ball it's worth taking the five seconds required to check that there are no nails or sharp edges sticking out. Tuck the ball behind you between your back and wall so that it pushes naturally into the curve of your spine. Be careful, however, not to try too

Here's an idea for you...

Fully aware of the benefits of weights for building both bone and muscle but just can't feel comfortable using dumbbells? Try combining dumbbells and the Swiss ball to increase the resistance of these exercises without the feeling of losing control. Perform any of these exercises as normal but with a dumbbell in each hand. Don't use anything too heavy at first (1 kg/2 pounds should be more than enough) until you have the feel for it and don't try to move the weights themselves – simply hold them in each hand, palms turned towards you, and pressed into your chest so they don't move around. Don't let the weights take your mind off your alignment. Remember the shoulder blades slide down (not yanked back), and don't forget to scoop that stomach and park that pelvis throughout the move. Try it, you'll like it.

hard to fit your shape to that of the ball – it's a ball, not even Raquel Welch was that curvy – as that can mean tipping your pelvis backwards in order to follow its curves. Although the ball is there to comfort and support you it should never tempt you into losing your neutral position. Just put the ball in place and park in neutral as you would if it wasn't there. Make sure your feet are hip-width apart and flat on the floor, with the knees very slightly bent. The feet should be placed a good foot length or more ahead of you so that as you bend your legs the kneecaps do not go further forward than your foot.

Slide your shoulder blades back and down, scoop your stomach, and breathing in, bend the knees and feel your back and ball moving down the wall. Don't go down so far that either your knees go further forward than your foot, or your bum drops lower than your knees. Now exhale and move back up to the start point, feeling the pressure in your thigh muscles. Make sure you resist the temptation to lock the knees at the top of the movement. Feel how smooth the movement is thanks to the ball, and how much easier it is than the same move without the ball which is now taking the weight and supporting you. Make sure you take equally long on both the upwards and downwards movement because they are both strength builders but for different muscles.

Enjoy the way that ball makes strength work seem more relaxing and even fun? Then turn to IDEA 30, *On the ball II*, to learn more.

Try another idea...

Essentially this move is a squat, an ugly name for what is considered the king of leg exercises because it works the calves, the hamstrings that flex the knee, the thighs (quads) that push upwards, the bum (glutes) and the back. Six repetitions will suffice unto the day.

There are a number of variations on this move, including the dancer's squat, and the ever so slightly less delicate sounding sumo squat.

DANCER'S SQUAT

As above except that you have your ankles closer together and the toes pointing apart in what dancers call a small turnout. Don't even think about trying this unless you are sure you know how to turnout (from the hips, remember) and even if you think you're sure why not take a quick look at IDEA 14, *Playing footsie*, just to be entirely sure. Six repetitions should be enough to prepare you for *Swan Lake*.

'The squat happens to be the single most effective exercise there is. Nothing else even comes close in terms of effectiveness, variety or metabolism-boosting ability.'
JEFF O'CONNELL, writing in
Men's Fitness

Defining idea...

SUMO SQUAT

If you are (or like to see yourself) as more of a ballerina than a bricklayer, then think of this as a plié. Begin as for the normal squat but with the feet placed slightly wider than shoulder-width and the toes pointed very slightly outwards. Think about the position and you'll see that the wider the legs, the more you resemble a sumo wrestler. Don't try to place your legs too wide at first, however, or you'll do yourself a mischief. (Unless, dear reader, you actually happen to be a sumo wrestler, in which case go for it.) The key difference with this variation is that it brings into play the muscles of the inner thighs (the adductors) as you push upwards and in doing so slightly close the legs. If you haven't worked those in a while you'll find out very quickly, so be gentle with yourself. Six repetitions, as ever.

How did it go?

Q **I know this sounds funny but I get lower back twinges even though the ball feels like it's supporting me perfectly. Why?**

A *It could be that your own muscles are pulling unevenly on your back. If your hip flexors are too tight, then they will have that effect. Take a look at IDEA 43, So hip it hurts, and make sure your hip flexors are properly stretched before you attempt squats.*

Q **Why does the ball try to escape up over my neck as I slide down?**

A *Either you're not so much sliding as diving like a footballer in the box, or else you're starting with the ball way too high up your back. Try starting with the ball in the middle of your back and slow the movement down.*

25

Foetal attraction

Rolling like a ball is one of the first exercises you encountered and still one of the best. If you enjoy curling into a ball there are lots of other ways to rock and roll.

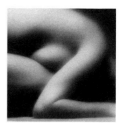

Rolling like a ball is such a pleasant way of unwinding that I can't understand why everyone doesn't do it as a simple trick to combat stress and stretch out the spine.

Mind you, that could be because my own natural reaction to pressure is to assume the foetal position and whimper. Turning that into a Pilates move came naturally. If you're comfortable with the basic roll, then there are a number of more elaborate variations based on the idea of rolling up backwards and forwards.

Just to recap, the basic roll, like a ball move, starts in the sitting position with the feet flat on the floor. Take hold of your shins with your hands and round out your back as if your whole spine was wheel-shaped. Keep your heels in to your hips and tip backwards so that you roll as far as your shoulders. Take care not to overdo it and roll onto your neck. To roll back, some instructors tell you to pull downwards with your hands on your shins but I was always told to initiate the movement with your stomach muscles and if you're comfortable with that, then I find it better for

Here's an idea for you...

Try the crab. Start sitting and pull your legs up to your chest, ankles crossed and knees wide. Reaching around the outside of your thighs, take left foot in right hand, right foot in left hand, and pull your legs towards your chest. Your feet should be right off the ground and your knees should be striving to meet your shoulders. The head is curled forwards but keep that 'apple' pinned between chin and chest so as not to constrict your airway. The reason for pulling your feet right in becomes clear on the forward part of the roll. As with the other rolls you inhale as you roll backwards as far as your shoulders so as to protect the neck. Exhale as you roll forward and continue right over so you come gently to rest with the top of your head touching the mat. If you imagine for a minute what happens to your head if you do this fast and fecklessly I'm sure you'll understand the need for gentleness and total control. Repeat six times.

encouraging that body consciousness (and keeping the stomach tensed). You should be able to roll smoothly, but with control, so that, for example, as you roll back up you can use your stomach muscles to stop yourself just before your feet return to the ground. Ten rolls followed by a full-length stretch on the floor (try to make yourself longer) should leave you feeling relaxed and ready to take on the world again.

The next step if you're on a roll is the seal – so named not because seals have a habit of grabbing their finny feet and rolling backwards, but because of the two claps that round off each repetition.

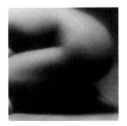

Starting in the sitting position, open your knees wide but press the soles of your feet together. Now reach down with your arms so that your elbows touch the inner thighs, your forearms are pressed into the calves of their respective legs, and your hands take hold of your ankles or instep. Joseph H.'s original move started off in a position with your feet about 10 cm (4 inches) off the floor, but as with many of his moves this has been modified by modern practitioners and some recommend starting with your feet, or just your toes, touching the ground (it's easier to balance and requires less effort from the stomach muscles). Curl your back into a perfect wheel shape, inhale and roll backwards as far as your shoulders. Hold your breath when you get there and 'clap' the soles of your feet together twice to finish off the move. This may seem strange but the idea is that it works your abs again by providing a bit of instability. Exhale as you roll back to your start position. Repeat six times.

If you're looking to roll away your stress by curling your spine, but don't have the luxury of being able to roll around on the floor like an oversized football, then take a look at **IDEA 23, *Backs against the wall*, for ideas on rolling your spine anytime, anyplace, anywhere.**

Try another idea...

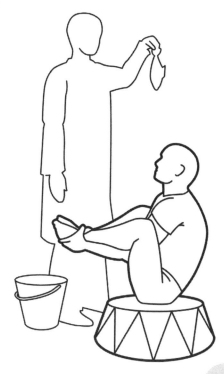

The Seal – *Joseph Pilates used to work in a circus. He must have been chuckling when he invented this one for us.*

Q I rolled backwards no problems, but simply can't roll back to where I started from. What am I doing wrong?

A *Are you sure you're holding your shins and not keeping your arms in to your body? If you're still having trouble you may need to work on your stomach muscles with the Hundred (see IDEA 20, Hundreds and thousands)*

Q I can roll backwards and return to the starting point but not to a point with my feet off the ground – instead the soles of my feet return to the ground with a slap. Why?

A *Are you sure you're using your stomach muscles to complete the roll, rather than relying on momentum to flip you back to where you started? Try slowing the move down further, and see if you can still return to the starting point, if you find you can't, then read the above.*

Defining idea...

'Let us roll our strength, and all our sweetness, up into one ball.'
ANDREW MARVELL

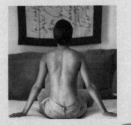

26

Let's twist again

Rotate to rejuvenate, work your waist, stretch your obliques and mobilise your spine. Go on, put a twist in your tail.

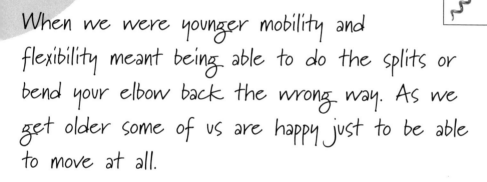

When we were younger mobility and flexibility meant being able to do the splits or bend your elbow back the wrong way. As we get older some of us are happy just to be able to move at all.

Mobility and flexibility are the key to staying young, avoiding injury and making the most of daily life, but they are the classic examples of the rule of 'use it or lose it'. You don't have to be a senior citizen to find that out. Spinal mobility is an issue for anyone who works at a keyboard. The good news is that you don't have to leave that keyboard to do something about it.

Seated on a chair, put your arms out straight, then bend them at the elbow so they cross in front of you like a Russian dancer with each hand flat, extended and parallel to the floor. One hand rests on top of the other elbow, the second hand is under the elbow of the first. Slide the shoulder blades back and down, and extend the neck as

Here's an idea for you... **Take a quick look at the illustration opposite. Obviously if you do start doing Pilates in the pub you run the risk of being stared at and possibly causing complete strangers to drop their crisps. Worse you could spill one of the glasses, which presumably isn't yours, and then all hell breaks loose. Don't say we didn't warn you. The idea of having a full glass (it doesn't have to be pint) in each hand, however, is a sure way of ensuring you're twisting smoothly and evenly, particularly if the glass happens to be full to the brim of precious liquid. If you do perform twists with anything in your hands, be particularly careful to slide your shoulder blades back and down. Otherwise you can end up using the shrugging muscles to help do the work and that creates tension in the neck. A slightly more common (but ultimately less fulfilling) prop is the simple pole or broom handle. Place the pole on the shoulders behind the back of the neck, with your elbow in front and beneath it and your wrists wrapped around so they rest on each end. You should look a little as if you'd been put in the stocks. Turning this way helps keep your arms and shoulders in line, and makes it much easier to feel the pivot at the hips and so keep the pelvis out of the movement.**

if that string was running through your spine and out the top of your head pulling you upwards. Scoop the stomach, park the pelvis and without moving the pelvis at all start breathing out, pivot the spine and head together slowly through 90 degrees so you are facing sideways. You should count five seconds to complete the move, breathing out smoothly all the while. Breathe in and return for the same count, then breathe out again and do the same to the other side. Six to ten twists to each side will help stretch and work the oblique muscles down the sides of your torso, and maintain the mobility of your spine while tensing the transversus for good measure. As an alternative you can extend the arms straight out to each side for the movement (be careful not to take out any desk lamps/potted plants/co-workers as you twist) to work the obliques a little harder and emphasise the movement. If you do that you will also add to the work done by the shoulders so it's important to ensure that they don't hunch up (see How did it go? below). Although it feels as if all of the work is being done by the upper body, this also brings in the lower body which is working unseen as it stabilises the pelvis to stop it from turning with your torso. By focusing on sliding the shoulders back it also helps open up the chest and encourages you to breathe deeply. All this means it can be a nifty little stress buster into the bargain. Ideally the move should be combined with some lateral stretching (see IDEA 27, *Lateral thinking*), to get all-round spine movement and stretch the muscles of the ribcage.

Having freed up your spine with a little rotation, it's time to get lateral and try some side bends. Take a look at IDEA 27, *Lateral thinking*, for more mobility and stretching.

Try another idea...

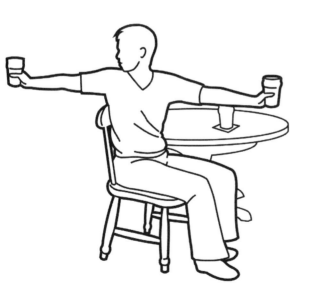

'You are old,' said the youth, 'as I mentioned before, And you have grown most uncommonly fat; Yet you turned a back-somersault in at the door Pray what is the reason for that?'
LEWIS CARROLL, Old Father William being clearly a man who takes his mobility and flexibility seriously

Defining idea...

Spinal twists, with a twist.
Smoothly does it, particularly if one of the pints isn't yours. Spillage may lead to IDEA 22, Take that!

How did
it go?

Q   It went just fine – what could I possibly be doing wrong?

A   Since you ask, try the move again and this time ask yourself whether your
shoulders are pulling up towards your head as you move. If so, you'll need
consciously to relax your trapezius muscle at the back of your neck and
slide the shoulder blades down. You might also be moving your head more,
or less, than your spine – it should move with the spine, balanced perfectly
on top without the neck itself twisting at all. Finally check that your pelvis
is stock still throughout the entire movement – the whole twist is in the
spine, not in the hips.

**Q   I can't turn through 90 degrees – I get stuck before then. Is this
bad?**

A   Only if it hurts. If it doesn't, then don't force the stretch, or try to 'bounce'
further round, but instead do the move smoothly and repeatedly each day
and you'll find that gradually you get more movement in the joint.

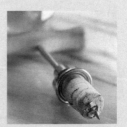

27

Lateral thinking

Whether we like it or not we spend all our upright day quietly compressing our spines and discs. No wonder we end the day slightly shorter than we started. So learn to stretch your sides and even stand tall – by bending over.

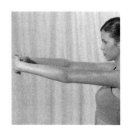

Dim memories of playing fields and school gyms have left a lot of us with the idea that warming up and stretching mean windmilling your arms a few times and maybe bouncing up and down a bit on the spot.

If we stretch at all it tends to be the big workhorse muscles of the limbs (see IDEA 7, *Workhorses and whippets*), and the large mobile joints such as the hips, knees and shoulders. We rarely spare a thought for the smaller muscles that help control poise and balance, let alone the less obvious joints, such as those between the vertebrae of the spine. Yet those smaller muscles and joints are key to core strength, and that means they're key to the Pilates concept of balance. Side stretches are a great way to gently work the whole of the side of your body from the shoulder to the hip.

Here's an idea for you...

If you really want to feel that stretch, then you'll need to find a pole. Don't be shy, get stretchy on the bus or train, wherever there's a pole you can grab hold of. The joy of poles is that you can grip them, and that in turn means that you can hold on to them and lean out further into the stretch. If you find a consenting pole, then take hold of it at the side but at arm's length (hard to do in a doorway). Feet together, stomach scooped and with a straight back, breathe out and stretch your other arm up in the air and slightly over your head as you lean away from the pole moving the weight towards the hip furthest from it (see illustration opposite). Count the five-second breath out and then return to upright. Don't forget to stretch both sides.

The working (or even non-working) day takes its toll in more ways than we are aware. The compression of the discs in the spine means it's not abnormal to be a centimetre shorter at the end of the day than you were when you woke up. That's not even taking into account the slump factor as tiredness causes us to lose our grip on posture. Stretching your spine may not suddenly expand those discs, but it reminds you of how tall you should be, and it wakes up all the muscles of the chest and back, including the intercostals that power so much of your breathing.

You don't have to have a prop to side stretch – you can simply stand tall in true Pilates style (pelvis parked, stomach scooped) and take one arm straight up and over your head before bringing it further over the top towards the other shoulder so you feel the stretch in your ribs. It's much more effective, however, to stretch with the aid of a prop – in this case the humble doorframe.

Stand feet-together in a doorframe far enough away from the right-hand side of it that you can bend your right arm 90 degrees at the elbow and place your hand on the doorframe round about the level of your waist. Now reach over the top of your head with your left hand and place that on the doorframe a little above your head. Breathe out and stretch your body away from the doorframe without moving either of your hands. Gently push the left hip away from the frame and feel that stretch through the intercostal muscles in your ribs and the muscles that run round the outside of your buttocks and down to the knee. Breathe out for

If stretching out your torso is floating your boat, then find out what the Swiss ball can do for you in IDEA 29, *On the ball I*.

Try another idea...

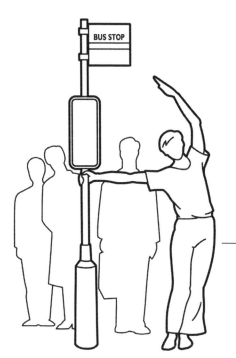

'*Each of us should do something every day That we do not want to do But we know we should do, To strengthen our backbone And put iron in our soul.*'
HENRY HITT CRANE, Methodist minister

Defining idea...

Singing in the rain?
While you're waiting why not ease into a lateral stretch? Ensure pole is firmly rooted or this may suddenly turn into mat work without the mat.

a slow count of five and then return to upright. Now stretch the other side for a count of five. Repeat that from four to six times per side for a full stretch. Notice that if you turn your armpit slightly up toward the ceiling you will also feel the stretch run right down your back through the latissimus dorsi ('lats') – the big triangular shaped muscles that form a line from your shoulders towards the small of your back.

How did it go?

Q   When I bend like you say, I get a pain in my lower back. How can I prevent that?

A   *First of all check your posture. While you are meant to be flexing your spine to the side that doesn't mean that it should be arching at all. Seen from the side your spine should still be normally aligned (see IDEA 8, Post office Pilates).*

Q   Feels great, but my consenting pole isn't in front of a mirror. Is there anything I might not be doing perfectly?

A   *Aside from arching the back, are you making sure that you're getting the stretch by pushing out towards the far hip, and not by squashing your ribs downwards on the near side to the pole? It is, after all, a stretch, not a scrunch.*

28

What the Feldenkrais!?

Pilates is an excellent means of re-educating your body to find perfect form and ease pain, but there are a number of other complementary techniques that may help you find out where the problem started in the first place.

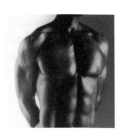

One of the purposes of Pilates is to correct your physical alignment and iron out all the kinks that life has put in.

Whether you tilt backwards through years of balancing the forward tilt of high heels, or slump your shoulders through a badly set-up keyboard, Pilates can help rejuvenate your body by literally setting you straight. Working out exactly where those imbalances are, however, is not necessarily part of the standard Pilates toolbox, and while there are Pilates experts who also have the skills to diagnose your imbalances, that is not always the case. For those times when conventional medicine or physiotherapy haven't hit the spot, it's worth knowing that there are other techniques that can come to your aid.

FELDENKRAIS: YOU WHAT!?

Where Pilates can be said to be strength through education, the Feldenkrais method is more about learning to focus on your own movements and positioning to re-educate your body to move differently.

To find out more about the Feldenkrais method, go to www.feldenkrais.com and choose the 'more Feldenkrais Method sites' button which allows you to choose from practitioners all over the world and find a class or teacher near you.

Dr Moshe Feldenkrais (1904–1984) was a judo black belt who spent his life studying patterns of movement, not least injured movement – an interest that had more than a little to do with his own crocked knee. Despite his own martial arts background, the doctor's technique is notably gentle, combining smooth movements and soft stretching, and is thereby perfect for those already suffering chronic pain (who might not therefore be ready for Pilates). As a re-education process it is not about trying to find a 'cure' for an illness, but instead about working out how to move smarter in daily life. Even the smallest of gestures has implications for bones, balance and brain, and the Feldenkrais method is all about awareness of how you move, and finding ways to make that easier. There are two main ways of conducting a Feldenkrais session: a group class called Awareness Through Movement®, and a one-on-one approach called Functional Integration®.

Awareness Through Movement is a class taking from half an hour to an hour, in which an instructor talks you through a series of movements that could be sitting, lying or standing. There are hundreds if not thousands of alternative series that may be practised and each one focuses on one area of movement.

As the good doctor himself puts it:

If Feldenkrais doesn't grab you, have a look at IDEA 34, *Yogalates*.

Try another idea...

'I begin by asking people to lie on their backs (after the same principle of reducing gravity) and learn to scan themselves. That is, they examine attentively the contact of their bodies with the floor and gradually learn to detect considerable differences – points where the contact is feeble or non-existent and others where it is full and distinct. This training develops awareness of the location of muscles producing weak contact through permanent excessive tension, thus holding parts of the body up off the floor...'

By talking a class through what it is they are feeling, the Feldenkrais method aims to increase awareness of how individuals perform individual movements. The gentleness is part of the technique – it's not just about avoiding pain for those who have it, the aim is never to stretch people to the limit so that 'pupils have the sensation of being able to do better, which induces more progress'.

The promises held out by this technique are nothing short of remarkable. The good doctor himself claimed that in some cases results can be obtained in only 20 minutes. So why not just try the technique? A single class is unlikely to break the bank or take too much out of your schedule and for many converts it has proved its worth on the spot.

'Make the impossible possible, the possible easy, and the easy elegant.'
Dr MOSHE FELDENKRAIS

Defining idea...

The other part of the method is a system of one-on-one sessions called 'functional integration', which usually involves lying on a therapy table. The instructor will take you through specific moves, but whereas group classes are entirely voice guided, the functional integration sessions are done by touch. Don't confuse this with massage, osteopathy or chiropractics, the idea is still about self-education and the touch is to help you focus on the muscles involved. It is not about healing or massaging the knots out of any part of you. Don't worry too much about the personal nature of touch either, the practitioners are very aware of the potential pitfalls of intimate contact and it is part of a code of practice that they will not touch you anywhere that is, ahem, delicate. Unlike sessions with the masseur or osteopath, the functional integration sessions are conducted fully clothed, which may come as a bit of a relief.

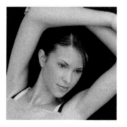 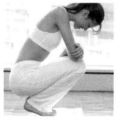 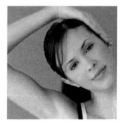

Q   **I went to a group class and learnt a lot about the way that I sit. How do I stop myself from going straight back to sitting the way I always did once I find myself in a chair?**

How did it go?

A   *Re-education is not an overnight process, especially when the thing you are trying to unlearn is a pattern built up over years if not decades. Dr Feldenkrais believed that the answer was to approach the action with many different exercises (rather than a few repeated over and over) and so you may need more than just one session to get a result. If it's a specific worry or niggle you have, then call up the centre and ask to speak to a practitioner in person to see what they suggest – you might want to try a one-on-one session.*

Q   **Is there an alternative to the classes? I can't make it at the regular times.**

A   *Feldenkrais is very much about the technique of talking you through the session and as a result the best way of doing it if you can't make it to a session is to buy one of the many audio tapes that are available. Try putting some gentle music on the CD and playing the tape (on a separate tape player) for a soothing session.*

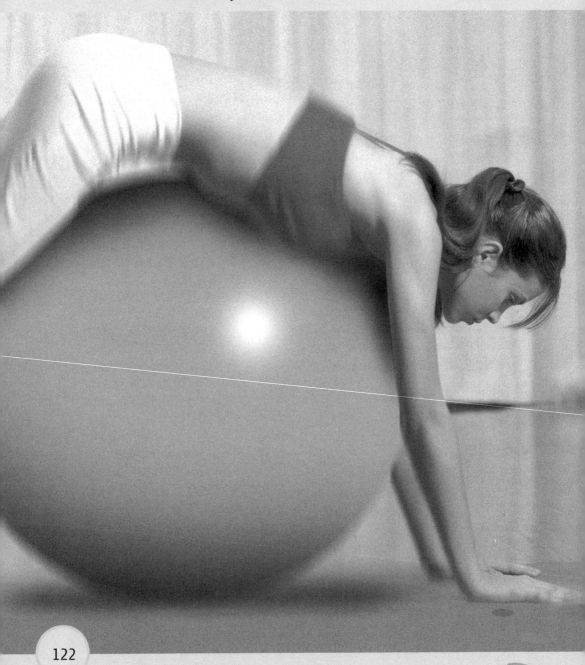

29

On the ball I: Stretches

Joseph H. Pilates never advocated the Swiss ball as part of the official equipment...but that's because he was born too soon to know the bliss of rainbow-coloured vinyl heaven.

Of all the many variants of Pilates that have popped up since Joseph H. popped his clogs, Pilates on the ball has proved one of the most popular.

It really doesn't take long to see why, in fact if you don't know why I can only think you've never had a chance to work with the Swiss ball. Swiss balls are just great. They're fun, they're colourful, they're soft, they're supportive and they're subtly challenging when it comes to core strength. Oh yes, and they even smell nice too. When it comes to Pilates they have two main roles. The first is to bring a whole new twist to old favourites with a different range of movements that can make you re-evaluate your technique. The other is to introduce entirely new moves to the mat work menu which make your routine less, well, routine.

If you're going to buy a Swiss ball be aware that not all balls are equal – they come in different diameters to suit different sized people. The key is being able to sit comfortably on top of the ball with your knees bent and your feet flat on the floor.

Go back to the back stretch on the ball and get into that position. Remember to scoop the stomach and park the pelvis which may mean lifting your buttocks up a bit to get it in line. Normally at this point you would have both feet flat on the floor to aid stability, but this time draw one foot back towards the ball. You will need to bend at the knee and the ankle will lift off the ground – that's fine, let it do so. Bring the foot in as close to the ball as you can, and drop the knee as far as it'll go. Now feel the stretch down the muscle of the front of your thigh (the quadriceps). Ease the leg back to the starting point and switch position to the other leg to stretch them both out.

Roughly speaking, a 45 cm ball suits people 1.40–1.52 m (4 feet 7 inches – 5 feet in old money), 55 cm balls are for those 1.55–1.68 m (5 feet 1 inch–5 feet 6 inches), and 65 cm for people who are 1.69–1.80 m (5 feet 7 inches–5 feet 11 inches). There are 75 cm balls for the six-footers (1.83 m) and even an 85 cm ball for basketballers, but you'll probably have to buy one from the US. The balls are tougher than you think and can take a full-grown man and all the weight he can heft on a pair of dumbbells. Although you can burst them if you press them onto something sharp, they don't explode, but just deflate pathetically, so don't be afraid to bounce on them. Just be careful you haven't left anything sharp lying around before you do.

When it comes to stretches and strength work (see IDEA 30, *On the ball II*) the ball has one outstanding feature. However comfortable the ball may seem, it is always inherently unstable, which means that whenever you trust your body to it you are having to do the stabilising yourself. That means subtly but constantly working all the balancing muscles of the body. It's perfect for building core strength, and for favouring the whippet muscles over the workhorses. At the same time the ball is soft and supportive, so as you drape yourself over it you can relax and stretch out, often achieving a deeper, longer stretch as a result.

BACK STRETCH

Try the back stretch for a start to get a feel for it. Sit on the centre of the ball, making sure that your feet are flat on the floor and a little apart to keep you rock solid and stable. Then very gently walk your feet away so that you lie back – don't worry: the ball will roll under you so that your back and neck come to be supported. You may want to have a hand behind your head to take the weight off your neck until it is resting on the ball. Try to lift your pelvis up so that it is in neutral, rather than flopping over backwards. If you focus on that you will realise that you are making lots of small movements to achieve that neutral position, and that's the essence of ball work. Now open up the arms crucifix style to fully open the chest and practice your deep and wide breathing. How good does that feel after a day bent over a sink or desk?

Balls aren't just for stretching – they're also for strength. See IDEA 30, _On the ball II_, for more about that.

Try another idea...

SIDE STRETCH

Kneel with the ball next to you and your arm resting on it. Now with the leg that's furthest from the ball, stretch straight out sideways and gently shift the weight onto the ball so you are completely draped over it sideways on. The hand that's not on the ball should now stretch up and over your head towards the ball. The hand that was resting on the ball can now rest on the floor on the other side of the ball so the curve of the ball completely fills the space between arm, armpit, ribs, hips and thighs. Scoop the stomach and make sure that your pelvis is parked (as seen side on). Feel the stretch in the side that's off the ball.

'i like my body when it is with your body. It is so quite new a thing.
**Muscles better and nerves more.'**
e. e. cummings, voicing a feeling many feel when working with another, even if it is only a Swiss ball.

Defining idea...

125

How did it go?

Q **I tried the thigh stretch on the ball but couldn't feel it – all I feel is that I am wobbling around a lot when I draw my foot back. How do I avoid that?**

A *What's happening is that when you move one foot back off the floor you destabilise yourself and your core muscles aren't yet used to re-establishing balance. Because you're still contending with that you aren't relaxing enough to fully draw back the foot and drop the knee enough to feel the thigh stretch. Don't worry, it will come (and in the meantime think of the good you're doing as you work your stomach muscles).*

Q **The back stretch feels divine but I'm not sure I'm using any muscles to balance. How can I feel that?**

A *Try shutting your eyes as you sit on the ball and then walk your legs away so you're lying down on it – you may feel a lot more of the balance going on.*

30

On the ball II: Strength work

The Swiss Ball can transform even the most familiar exercise into a new workout challenge. Here are some strength exercises given a makeover with the great globe of fun.

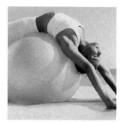

Joseph Pilates would have just loved the Swiss ball for strength exercises.

Its basic instability means that any strength work done resting on it automatically recruits so many more of the muscles that contribute to core strength. It brings a whole new dimension even to such old favourites as the press-up, making what is normally a chest exercise into a whole-body workout with infinite gradations of difficulty.

PRESS-UPS ON THE BALL

The standard press-up (see IDEA 15, *Drop and give me twenty*) is a move that demands hard work from the chest, shoulders and the back of the arm. It's a classic and a great strength move, but for a lot of people it's deeply off-putting and not just because of its hard-man image. For a start it's simply too hard for many of us, and secondly the arms and chest are the muscles men tend to want to tone up, women are usually less interested. By taking the press-up onto the ball, however, there is a major shift in emphasis. Now the lower body is supported by the ball, which is

Here's an idea for you...

If you're confident that you can perform the press-up with good form, then why not go one step further and try the full pike? This move takes away the emphasis on the chest and instead shifts the workload to the abdominals. Depending on your bodyweight you may also find that it puts a lot of load on your shoulders.

Start as for the press-up by kneeling in front of the ball, then lying over it and finally walking the hands away until the ball is down by your ankles and your arms are taking your weight with your hands spread on the floor shoulder-width apart. Now breathe out and roll the ball up with your feet until you are in the pike position – your pelvis is lifted right up, and your weight is tipped forward onto your shoulders as the line of your back goes up to as close to vertical as you can comfortably manage. This is not an exercise for the faint hearted or those with flabby abs as the amount of torso tensing needed to maintain balance is considerable. Five seconds breathing out as you pike, hold it for a moment, and then inhale as you go back to the press-up position. As for repetitions, I refer you to Joseph's original press-up recommendation of three and no more.

always about to make a bid for freedom. That puts much more stress on the buttocks and back to keep straight, and on the stomach muscles and obliques to counter the small but non-stop wobbles. Which means that while it still tones up the torso, it's also a great tum toner. Which in turn broadens its appeal.

Kneel in front of the ball and roll your upper body onto and over it until your arms can reach down the other side to place the palms of your hands on the floor. Now walk forwards with your hands so that the ball rolls further down your body. How far you go is up to you. The further down your legs the ball is, the more weight your chest and shoulders will have to take, so if you're feeling strong it can be by your ankles but if not it could be on your upper thighs. Because there are an infinite number of subtly graded positions between these two extremes, the ball makes it possible gradually to increase your workload over time.

When you have your preferred position, think about finding neutral and scooping your stomach before breathing out, bending your elbows and lowering your chest towards the floor for a count of five. Then breathe out and straighten the arms to push back to where you started, also for a count of five. Don't lock your elbows at the top of the movement. Joseph Pilates originally recommended three press-ups as all you needed to do, but if you're feeling more comfortable, and particularly if you're not pressing your full weight, then you may want to do anywhere from five to ten. Do remember it's about quality not quantity.

Much of the effort of these exercises consists of the abs battling the ball's urge to roll away. A different take, and one that is particularly good for the obliques, is to battle gravity with static work – see IDEA 26, *Let's twist again.*

Try another idea...

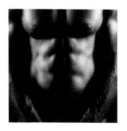

'Anatomy is destiny.'
SIGMUND FREUD

Defining idea...

Q **I like the ball but I'm very wobbly and expend so much effort balancing that I can barely perform a single press-up. How can I work on that?**

A   *Try doing some of the easier exercises first until you are more at ease on the ball. If you try doing side twists (see IDEA 26, Let's twist again) seated on the ball, for example, you'll get more used to the way it moves.*

Q **I like the idea of the pike but just can't get my back anywhere near vertical. Is there a way of making it easier?**

A   *Yes, don't focus on trying to get vertical at all. Simply aim to lift your pelvis higher than your abs and hold it there. Instead of working on raising yourself higher, work on being more stable for longer in the lower position. See if you can practice 'wide' breathing while you're there. Once you have that mastered you'll be able to lift the pelvis much higher.*

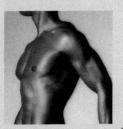

31
Your flexible friend I: Toning up topside

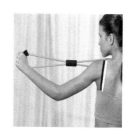

You've been playing with rubber bands since you were a kid. Now learn how to perfect your poise and power as you play with them the grown-up way.

Resistance bands are those glorified giant rubber bands either sold in loops or by the metre from sports shops and Pilates studios.

They may not be much to look at but they are just fabulous for a number of reasons:

- They're incredibly versatile – whether you want to work limbs or develop core strength.
- You can adjust the difficulty as subtly as you wish by shifting your grip.
- They're just as good for stretching as for strength building.
- You can slip them in your pocket and take them on business trips or on holiday.
- They cost less than lunch from a sandwich bar.
- They come in different degrees of resistance (stretchiness) so you can easily progress from easier to harder.

Here's an idea for you... If you're feeling strong enough to try the press-ups in IDEA 15, *Drop and give me twenty*, then here's a way of using the rubber band to add a little extra spring to the movement. It's especially useful if you find box press-ups (on your knees) a little too easy but aren't comfortable with the full-length version. This way you can do box press-ups but make the resistance a little harder. Kneel on the floor with the band around the back of your shoulders like a shawl – one end in each hand. Now stretch your arms out forwards and drop down onto your hands into the press-up position. As you breathe in, bend your elbows and lower yourself towards the floor, the band relaxes. As you breathe out, however, and straighten your arms to straighten up again, you are stretching the band which adds its resistance to your bodyweight to make the movement harder. Four to six press-ups, counting five on each breath, should be fine.

I love resistance bands: come to think of it, what with that and my unnatural enthusiasm for the Swiss ball, I'm well on my way to full-blown rubber fetishism.

Joseph H. was born too young to include resistance bands when he first developed his theories of Pilates but they are entirely in line with the principles of steady resistance that he built into such machines as the Pedipull. Bands have the added benefit that they cost a fraction of a full resistance machine and take up no space whatsoever for when you're on the road or if you fancy having a gym in your pocket at work. The following are some ideas for exercises to help tone the upper body; for more exercises focusing on the lower body, take a look at IDEA 32, *Your flexible friend II.*

GETTING FIT WHILE YOU SIT

All of these exercises can be done while sat in a chair. Remember to keep both feet flat on the ground for stability, to lengthen the neck and spine as if being pulled up on a string and to park the pelvis and scoop the stomach.

Triceps

Start with the band held in both hands, arms up in the air. Now take one arm down to the side (you'll find you have to twist the wrist in the process to accommodate the band) so that the arm that is left up has to bend at the elbow. One hand should now be at your side,

If you like the idea of strength work to tone your body, take a look at IDEA 32, *Your flexible friend II*, and see how the resistance band can help work your lower body too.

Try another idea...

the other resting behind your head with the band tight (depending on your degree of strength) between the two. Now without moving any other part of your arm or shoulder simply straighten the bent arm at the elbow so the hand moves away from your head. You should feel the resistance in the triceps muscle which runs down the back of your arm and straightens it. Remember to breathe out as you straighten for a count of five, and then in as you return, equally slowly to your starting point. Six repetitions and then change sides to do the other arm.

Biceps

Place one end of the band on the floor pinned down by something sturdy – your foot should do the job. Sitting down, lean forward slightly to reach for the band with one hand. Your elbow should rest on the inside of your thigh just above the knee. Now with the band wrapped around the knuckles of your fist breathe out and bend the elbow for a count of five so your fist comes right up to your shoulder. Breathe in and return just as slowly to the starting point. Change arms after six repetitions and repeat with the other arm.

'The path of least resistance is the path of the loser.'
H. G. WELLS

Defining idea...

Here's an idea for you...

Chest

Remember when chest expanders were the last word in home gyms? The adverts featured complicated combinations of springs and/or sprung poles being manipulated by huge muscly men. Well this is the same kind of thing without the hassle or expense. Simply hold your arms out in front of you with the band stretched between the two hands. Keep the elbows very slightly bent and open your arms to bring your hands back nearly in line with your shoulders. Try not to bring your elbows back further than your shoulders or you risk straining the front of your shoulder muscle. This should open up your chest perfectly as you breathe out for a five count on opening the arms, and in for a five count as you return them to the start position in front of you. Remember Joseph Pilates' advice to completely empty the lungs as you breathe. Don't forget to keep your spine in neutral at all times.

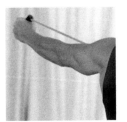 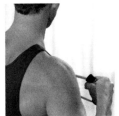

Q   I'm finding it too easy to stretch the band however short I make it. Is there any way of making this harder?

How did it go?

A   *Certainly, resistance bands come in different strengths, normally colour coded so you can see which is which. If your local sports shop only stocks the easier, more stretchy ones, then find a Pilates studio or enquire at a physiotherapists where they will have the stronger bands used in rehabilitation.*

Q   I like the idea of the resistance-added press-up but hate press-ups. How can I work the muscles without getting down and dirty?

A   *Work on the chest press first by putting the band around your back and then, holding an end in each hand, extend your arms straight out forwards. Remember not to lock the elbow.*

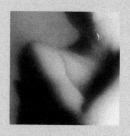

135

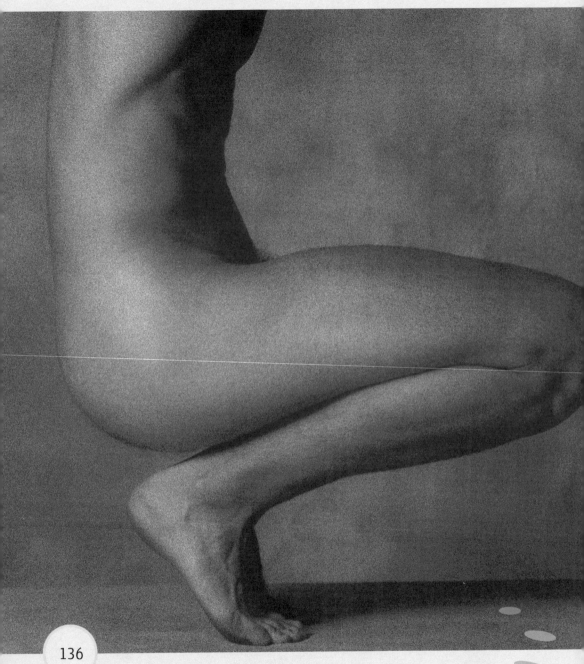

32

Your flexible friend II: Long, lean legs

In IDEA 31, *Flexible friend I*, you saw how an oversized rubber band can help tone muscle above the waist. Here's how our stretchy friend can help you develop long, lean legs.

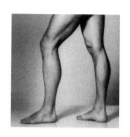

Resistance bands are just great for a Pilates approach to strength because they apply a constant resistance just like cable machines (see Idea 18, 'Man and machine', for more on that).

They offer many of the same benefits of weights, including building strength and fighting osteoporosis, but unlike weights you can't drop them, they aren't lumpy and ugly, they don't make clanking noises at home and you can pack them away in a pocket. They do have one potential pitfall though: they ping like anyone's business if you let go of one end. To do the major leg muscle exercises shown here it's very important to have the band firmly secured at the other end so it can't snap back and cause havoc. For that you may want either to invest in a very long strip of band so you can tie one end to a handle/piece of furniture, or else make sure you buy a loop so you can loop it around handles, etc. As well as the original resistance

Here's an idea for you... **Another way to use the band to tone the top of your thighs is to lie on the mat on your back with your feet flat on the floor and a looped band around your bent knees. If you now breathe out and open your knees as widely as you can for a count of five, then breathe in as you bring them back to the start point, you'll also work those abductors.**

bands there are also resistance cords which are much the same but have the advantage of handles. Some people find these easier to use, others find them less adaptable to different exercises. You pays your money...

With workhorse muscles of the thighs, hamstring and bum (glutes) tending to do most of the work of getting us around, it's easy to ignore the abductor and adductor muscles that open and close the thighs. Usually we don't really know they're there until we do something unusual (like dancing, playing football, hopscotch or skipping sideways) after which they will feel tender. Strengthening them avoids that, helps strengthen the legs and tones the tops of the thighs.

STANDING ADDUCTOR EXERCISE

With one end of the band firmly secured, stand sideways on to the anchor point with the other end of the band looped around the ankle of the leg nearest the anchor. 'Turn out' the leg with the loop in ballet fashion, so that the leg turns outwards from the hip to point the toes away from the body. Now keeping the leg absolutely straight, pull the ankle towards the supporting leg (furthest from the anchor point). This should mean that the adductor muscle (inside top of the thigh) that closes the thighs is now working against the band. Ten repetitions breathing out to pull against the band for a count of five, and in to return to the start position for a count of five. Repeat with the other leg. Don't forget the scooped stomach and parked pelvis.

STANDING ABDUCTOR EXERCISE

Have the band anchored as before but this
time looped around the ankle furthest from
the anchor point. Once again the leg is turned
out ballerina style and this time the exercise consists of opening the turned out leg,
pulling it away from the supporting leg so that it stretches the band to open and
relaxes it to return. Breathing and repetitions as before. Abduction (moving away
from the body's centre line) works the muscles around the top of the outside of the
thigh.

**If you want to work the smaller
muscles of the calf, shin, ankle
and feet, then take a look at
IDEA 14, *Playing footsie.***

*Try
another
idea...*

FOOT AND ANKLE EXERCISES

Simply sit in a chair with your leg stretched out in front of you (taking care not to
lock the knee) and a long loop of band looped around the ball of your foot and held
in your hand so that you are pulling the ball of your foot back towards you.
Without moving at the knee, stretch the band further by pointing the foot away
from you. This exercise strengthens the ankle joint and the calf muscles.

Now move the band to the toes and this time point the toes against the resistance
of the band. This strengthens the toes and tendons and can help avoid injury
among runners and dancers who may be light on their feet but still put their
tootsies through tough times.

**'Ankles are nearly always
neat and good-looking, but
knees are nearly always not.'**
DWIGHT D. EISENHOWER

*Defining
idea...*

ANKLE AND SHIN

Cross your right leg lightly over the lower part of the left leg so the right ankle is resting on the left shin. Now loop the band securely around the toes and the ball of the right foot. Hold the other end in your left hand so that you are pulling the toes back towards your left hand. Now flex the ankle so that the foot points upwards and away from your left hand, stretching the band as it does. You should feel this in the ankles and the muscles of the shin. Breathe out with the effort for a count of five and do six to ten repetitions for each foot.

How did it go?

Q   I'm happy to loop the band around my knees but find it very easy. Can't I work my thighs harder than that?

A   *OK, try looping the band around both knees and this time turning onto your side with your head resting on the hand of the arm on the ground and the other arm out, hand on the ground to steady you. Bend the knees at right angles and try to stretch the top one as far from the bottom one as possible. You will find this puts much more of a stretch into the top of your thigh.*

Q   I've tried the band and am getting a rash, why?

A   *It could be that you are sensitive to the rubbing, in which case simply do the exercises wearing leggings or tights (especially if you have hairy legs). It is also possible that you are allergic to latex. Try a non-latex band (they smell better too).*

33

In a spin – Gyrokinesis

Interested in the crossover between dance and yoga? Or maybe you've seen the term Gyrokinesis among the classes at your Pilates studio and wondered what it is. Either way, read on.

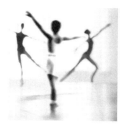

Gyrokinesis (literally a rotating movement) is a system of 'yoga for dancers' and one of the most recent yoga/dance hybrids to be presented in Pilates studios.

Gyrokinesis is the brainchild of Juliu Horvath, who was a classical dancer with the Romanian State Opera. Making a career move in more ways than one, he defected and danced in New York and with the Houston Ballet before a torn Achilles tendon effectively ended his dancing days. Horvath turned to yoga, and in particular kundalini yoga, as both consolation and rehabilitation, and developed his own system of moves. Kundalini yoga takes as its starting point the idea that there is an enormous reserve of untapped potential residing in all of us like a coiled snake at the base of the spine. Gyrokinesis too takes the spine as the focal point of power and movement, but blends in more Western ideas of movement and exercise from dance to gymnastics.

Here's an idea for you... **Fancy the sound of Gyrokinesis but there's no practitioner near you? There probably is but they may be cunningly camouflaged as a Pilates studio. Gyrokinesis is commonly practised alongside mainstream Pilates. To find out which studios offer it, go to www.gyrotonic.com where there is a finder of coaches and studios.**

Like Pilates, the system has a series of core moves aimed at mobilising the spine (but using small stools rather than mat work) and has its own machines to take resistance movements further if students wish. Underlying the practice are seven essential elements of spinal movement including forwards, backwards, the left side, the right side, twists, circular rotations and smaller joint articulations. Classes start off with 'self-massage' and breathing exercises before going into dance-inspired curling, arching and spiralling moves where fluidity is the key. The aim is to stimulate the nervous system and give a wider range of movement to all of the joints while more advanced classes work on muscular endurance for more strenuous exercise.

The idea is that where traditional Western exercise tends to obsess about muscular development, Gyrokinesis focuses on the articulation of the joints and in particular on strengthening the ligaments that link bone to bone. That emphasis on joint strength has an obvious appeal to dancers and athletes, for whom the joints are often the weak point, but also for anyone who's ever suffered so much as a twinge in the knee.

Much like Pilates, Gyrokinesis offers both group classes with their staple exercises and a system of resistance moves done on specially designed machines. The machine work goes under the name of Gyrotonics® and uses weights, pulleys and wheels to set up spherical or spiral movements to work the joints along the principles of fluid movement laid down by the rest of the method. Flexibility in the spine and increased co-ordination are considered particularly important, and according to Horvath the moves are inspired by a cocktail of influences including yoga, tai-chi, dance and swimming. Like Pilates, the method talks of lengthening muscle rather than bulking it up, but unlike the teachings of Joseph H., Horvath makes much of the energy flowing along the meridian lines of the body.

If the idea of fusion fitness fires you up, then take a look at other East meets West techniques such as yogalates (see IDEA 34, *Yogalates*). If it's the idea of non-impact resistance training with machines that appeals, then try IDEA 36, *Rack and roll with the Reformer.*

Try another idea...

Fans call the Gyrotonic system the 'fitness machines of the future' and rave about the benefits of circular movements that are more ergonomically in tune with the mobility and articulation of the human body. Undoubtedly the principles are sound and if the sphere of movement is less linear, the concept behind the resistance machines is not so very different from those of Joseph H. – which is why the two systems so often co-exist in the same studio. On the downside the Gyrotonic machines are relatively rare, and correspondingly expensive, and since Mr Horvath has taken care to keep total control over the method (he alone supervises instruction of teachers), there isn't much chance of competition coming in to bring the prices down.

'It is not bulk that produces strength, it is the connections between the joints.'
JULIU HORVATH, who may sound uncommonly like a Klingon but does know a thing or two about tendons.

Defining idea...

143

Q I like the idea but I've never tried yoga and the closest I've come to dancing is pogoing to the Sex Pistols. Is there anything in it for me?

A *If you already practise Pilates, then the degree of dance and mysticism in Gyrokinesis is unlikely to be that much of a challenge. As for the benefits, there is a lot to be said for the emphasis on tendons (connecting muscle to bone) and ligaments (connecting bone to bone) which are often neglected despite being the weak point in many of our muscular movements. The smart option would be to try the group Gyrokinesis classes and not splash out on individual Gyrotonic sessions unless the value of the group work is clear in your case.*

Q I tried a class and liked the moves but those little stools – what a pain in the bum! What can I do?

A *The stools are part and patented parcel of the approach, so if you go to classes you'll have to use them. At home, however, you could always try some moves on the Swiss ball.*

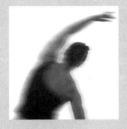

34

Yogalates

Yoga meets Pilates – result Yogalates. It sounds like something you'd order to go from a coffee bar but there are plenty who swear by it, which means it's popping up on the planner at a studio or gym near you.

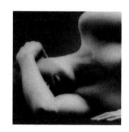

The fitness industry is appropriately hyperactive and so the arrival of Yogalates should come as no surprise.

After all, pretty much every other combination of exercise has been tried (Yoga Spinning® anyone?), and yoga and Pilates are more obviously complementary than most. So while waiting for someone to commercialise aqualates (it has to happen), why not try a taste of Yogilates®/Yogalates – the fusion fitness flavour of the moment.

If you're wondering about the two forms of spelling the answer is simple. Yogilates® was created in 1997 by a Pilates instructor and hatha yoga expert called Jonathan Urla. The story goes that he chanced upon the idea by taking one class after the other and appreciating that the Pilates work, in opening up his breathing and stretching out his body, had made him notably more receptive to the benefits of the yoga *asanas* (postures). He then blended the breathing of yoga and the core strengthening, alignment awareness and spine lengthening of Pilates mat work, and

Here's an idea for you...

The 'full cobra' is a great exercise for spine mobility, for arm strength, filling the lungs with (hopefully fresh) air, and above all for working the spinae erector muscles that run down the back and bend your backbone backwards.

Start face down on the mat with your elbows bent and your palms on the floor, fingers spread wide and fingertips roughly level with your shoulders. Breathe out and lift your chest and shoulders off the floor keeping your chin tucked in, pinning an imaginary apple between chin and chest. The effect of that is to open out the airways. Keep curling (think of one vertebrae at a time) backwards until you are raised as far as you can and let your head come up so you're looking forwards. Try not to move your elbows. Breathe widely and hold for 30 seconds or so before bending the elbows and curling back down again. Follow up with the 'resting child' (see IDEA 41, *Feelin' good*).

hatha yoga poses, before finishing off each and every Yogilates class with a relaxation technique called shavasana that stresses stillness and meditation. As is the way with these things, Urla promptly registered the idea, including the spelling and so anything Yogilates relates to his ideas. You can buy the Yogilates book and DVD from websites around the world, but at the time of writing true trademark Yogilates sessions are a tad tough to find outside of LA and New York.

Yogalates, on the other hand was the name chosen by an Australian Pilates expert, Louise Solomon, for her flavour of fusion, and along with the book and videos her classes are commonly found in Europe as well as Down Under.

Yogalates sessions pay particular attention to the core strength and spinal and pelvic awareness, as you'd expect from the Pilates lineage. Unlike Yogilates, Yogalates also makes much use of resistance bands (see IDEA 31, *Your flexible friend I*) to strengthen and stretch the muscles in the quest for balance. The yoga element comes in with a greater emphasis on breathing, with *pranayama* yogic breathing techniques being used alternately to energise and relax. Much as Yogilates ends with the *shavasana* session, Yogilates ends with a chanting of the Sanskrit phrase 'namaste' which is translated to mean 'the divine in me recognises the divine in you'. Well that's officially how it's translated. I'm reliably assured that in Nepal and India the phrase is so multipurpose that it can mean pretty much everything from 'hello' to 'two pints of lager and a packet of crisps please'. OK, maybe not that *reliably* assured, but assured anyway.

> **For a more detailed look at a combined Pilates/yoga move, go to IDEA 35, *Here comes the sun*, and learn about one move that can be found in pretty much every form of yoga/Pilates fusion. If the general idea of fusion takes your fancy, then take a look at IDEA 33, *In a spin*, and find out about Gyrokinesis.**
>
> *Try another idea...*

Purists sniff at fusion fitness, but then sniffing is what purists do best, and even cynics have to admit that Pilates and yoga do share a great deal in terms of goals and even some moves and techniques. Probably the best way to see it is that a fusion approach will offer more body toning than all but the most energetic forms of yoga (such as vikram) while it will focus more on breathing and calmness than pure Pilates. Overall, the joy of fusion is variety and fans will gush spontaneously about the feeling of well-being induced by a good session. And only a hardcore killjoy would argue with that.

> **'Relax, receive, and renew – this is the future of fitness!'**
> The promise of Yogilates
>
> *Defining idea...*

How did
it go?
Q **Should I feel so tight at the front of my shoulders?**

A *No, it sounds as if you are pushing very hard and lifting yourself with your triceps (the back of your arms) rather than using your arms to help you curl your spine back to raise the head and chest. Make sure you're not locking your elbows at the top of the move. If you keep your elbows soft you're less likely to tense up.*

Q **Tried the class. Liked it. Now how do I do it at home?**

A *Louise Solomon will be delighted you asked. There is a video or DVD of the same name, which is refreshingly straightforward.*

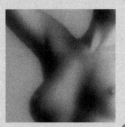

35

Here comes the sun...

Start the day by saluting the sun and add a pinch of paganism to your Pilates.

Time to come clean. I'm not exactly what you'd call a yoga expert. In fact when I hear the word 'yogi' I still think it refers to a 'smarter than average bear' who lives in Jellystone National Park.

However, I happen to love the sun salutation (that's *suryanamaskar* to its mates) not least because it brings an agreeable pinch of paganism to Pilates. Plus it's based on sun worshipping and if like me you're born and bred in the London drizzle, then sun worshipping is totally understandable in all its forms.

If you're wondering what a series of yoga *asanas* (positions) is doing in a book on Pilates, the answer is that while there are a variety of different yoga/Pilates fusions (see IDEA 34, *Yogalates*), one of the points they all have in common is that they include the sun salutation series. Why? Because it's fab, that's why.

To do it properly requires some supervised instruction, because breathing correctly and ensuring the fluid transition from one pose to the next is not a simple matter.

Although the beauty of the sun salutation series is the fact that it is a combo of quality moves, you may find them all a bit much to take in at once. Try breaking them down into their component parts to master them individually. For the 'downward facing dog', for example, you may find it easier to start in the 'resting child' position (see IDEA 41, *Feelin' good*) with your hands out in front of you, palms on the ground and elbows off the floor. Breathe out and come up onto all fours, then put the balls of your feet onto the ground and smoothly sway the hips upwards until you are resting on the balls of your feet and the palms of your hands. Pull your bellybutton towards your backbone (see IDEA 5, *Scoop!*) throughout. When you want to come out of the position again, push backwards so the weight moves more towards your heels (but see How did it go? below) and then bend the knees so that you come gently back to the floor and can go back into the 'resting child'.

The following can only be a rough guide to give you a general idea of the series that you will encounter in a Yogalates/Yogilates class and the breathing instructions have been simplified. As you try it you will very quickly realise that this combines a number of moves, any one of which would be a great way of toning up to face the day. Combined they're unbeatable. It's worth going to a class just to learn this series. Start standing with feet hip-width apart, knees very slightly bent, stomach scooped, pelvis parked and your arms by your sides. Breathe out and raise your arms at your sides, turning your palms up to the sky and bring them right up until they are straight up in the air as you greet the sun. Breathe in for a five count and then breathe out again, bending the knees and bringing the hands down as you bend gently down until you can place your fingertips alongside your toes on the floor. Breathe in again and extend the right foot back and place the bent right knee on the floor. Make sure your forward (left) knee doesn't extend beyond the foot (see IDEA 23, *Backs against the wall*). This should look like a classic sprinter's stretch, and guess what? It is. Now push the left leg right back to join the right and go up on the toes and straightened arms as if about to perform a press-up. Keep your back straight.

To help break the idea down take a look at IDEA 34, *Yogalates*, and its explanation of the 'full cobra' part of the move.

Try another idea...

Breathing in, drop both knees to the floor and arch the back down as you bend your arms and drop your chest to the floor as if you were doing a box press-up but have forgotten that your bum is still sticking up in the air. From there it's time to go into the 'full cobra' (body lying on floor, arms extended so head and chest rise up) as you breathe out. From the 'full cobra' place the soles of the feet on floor and push back and up, straightening the legs and walking back the hands until you're in the 'downward facing dog' (you should now look like an inverted V). Breathe in and bring the right foot forward to the hands and bend the knees so the left knee rests on the floor – this should be the partner move to the sprinter stretch you were in earlier. Again ensure your knee doesn't go past the foot. Now breathe out again and bring your other foot up to join the right and push up so that you are again bent over, hands on the floor, toes and fingers in line. Finally straighten up, arms rising at your sides until they are straight above your head.

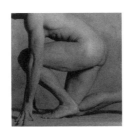

'**Both Yoga and Pilates were created with the belief that through disciplined practice, one cannot only develop tremendous physical skills and improve health, but can also transform oneself mentally and spiritually to a higher plane.**'
JONATHAN URLA

Defining idea...

Q   It went fine but when I get to the 'downward facing dog' part the muscles in the backs of my leg feel way too tight for comfort. Any ideas?

A   *Remember that you are not trying to plant your heels on the floor as you do this. Your hamstrings may be too tight to let you get near to that point (especially if you're a man) and it's not a required feature, so let your heels rise up to take the pressure off the back of your knees. As always in mat work, make sure that your knees don't lock out at any point during the series.*

Q   When I do the full cobra I feel stiff in my back. What can I do to help that?

A   *Are you doing any work to strengthen the erector spinae muscles of your back? If you're a relative beginner try the exercises in IDEA 23, Backs against the wall, and then move on to the stretches in IDEA 29, On the ball I, to ease out the stiffness of your back.*

152

36

Rack and roll with the Reformer

It looks and sounds like something straight out of the Inquisition, but don't be afraid – the Reformer is a great piece of kit for adding more resistance to familiar exercises.

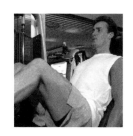

The Reformer was one of Joseph Pilates' first pieces of tailor-made equipment and it's hard not to see it as a direct descendant of the bed frame and bedspring contraptions he knocked up while interned in the war as a way of keeping his fellow inmates hale and hearty.

If its ancestry is apparent, however, so is the fact that the machine has come a long way since then.

The heart of the Reformer is a sliding platform big enough to rest your entire torso on. This platform can be propelled up or down the frame either by pushing with

Here's an idea for you...

Try doing the Hundred on the Reformer. Take a look at the illustration opposite and you'll see that the body position is exactly the same, with the legs in the air and the hands performing the air-slap to the sides. The difference is that instead of being completely free the hands are looped through straps leading to the top of the frame. These are providing resistance where ordinarily there is none, meaning that the body is having to push down with the shoulders and the lateral muscles of the back. As the arms pump the air they are pulling on the straps and therefore also pulling the body on the slide. Controlling the movement of the body adds to the amount of work being done by the abdominal and stabilising muscles and so increases the benefits for core stability.

the legs against a kick bar at the bottom of the frame, or by pulling on ropes attached at the top. Remember those 50s films where radiation caused spiders and other creepies to mutate into giant monsters? Well, if a traditional gym rowing machine were to be exposed to the same kind of radiation this is the monster it would turn into.

The whole point is that you can perform the Pilates exercises you are already familiar with from mat work, but with the twist that you now have to balance on a moving platform and control that movement against the resistance of springs. To add to the surprises the device can throw at you there is a system of springs, straps and pulleys that an instructor can combine to create over a hundred exercises to add variety and complexity. The springs are adjustable, so resistance is progressive, allowing users to gradually increase strength while lengthening the muscles. As with all other Pilates strength work, this is designed so as not to build bulk, so don't worry about turning all Arnie overnight. Most people's first reaction, after mild panic at the thought of being attached to what looks like a torturer's rack, is that the exercises seem exceedingly simple and easy. The slide of the Reformer is effortless and exercises are low or zero impact so you're encouraged to engage muscles without any of that 'no pain, no gain' rubbish that was so popular in the 80s.

If hardware seems to you to be the way to go to take your technique further, then the next major piece of Pilates kit after the Reformer is the Cadillac. To learn how to get behind the wheel, turn to IDEA 39, *Cruising in the Cadillac*.

Try another idea...

At a slight disadvantage.
Please note, it is recommended to check at this point if this man is a qualified Pilates practitioner. If not you want to get the law on him pronto.

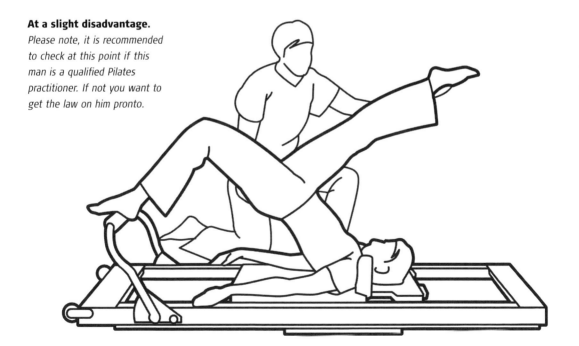

155

'It is a dangerous thing to reform anyone.'
OSCAR WILDE

In days gone by the Reformer was such an expensive item that studios rarely had more than one or two and all Reformer work was done as one-on-one tuition, which didn't come cheap. Now that Reformers are much more common, and cheaper versions have appeared on the market to cater for groups, it's not so rare to find studios and even gyms with dedicated Reformer rooms where you can be on the rack alongside half a dozen others. Just as group classes eased you into Pilates on the mat, you may find this the best way to experiment with taking your technique further. It's not the only way though. With more machines available it's becoming normal for instructors to take newcomers through their paces on a Reformer and then subsequently allow them to work on the machines on their own as it suits them. This all makes it an ideal way of pushing through a Pilates plateau, giving yourself a new challenge or simply trying something new for the sake of it.

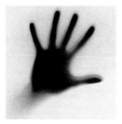
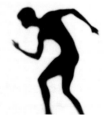

Q   **I tried a group session and found it very relaxing. Too relaxing actually – I really didn't feel that I was making any effort. Will I have got any benefit?**

How did it go?

A   *The whole Pilates approach avoids the received idea that if it didn't hurt you didn't do it hard enough, but if you're used to Pilates practice and didn't feel that the Reformer moves were adding anything, then you should say so to the instructor who may be willing to show you how to increase the resistance of the springs (for example) and let you practice on your own to see if you still feel that you're being sufficiently challenged.*

Q   **I tried the Hundred on the Reformer and my shoulders feel sore. What should I do?**

A   *That's because the deltoid muscle of the shoulder is now being brought into play because of the hand loops. Have a word with your instructor but as an interim move you may want to bend your elbows a little more at the beginning of the move so that the push down comes partly from the triceps as they straighten your arms.*

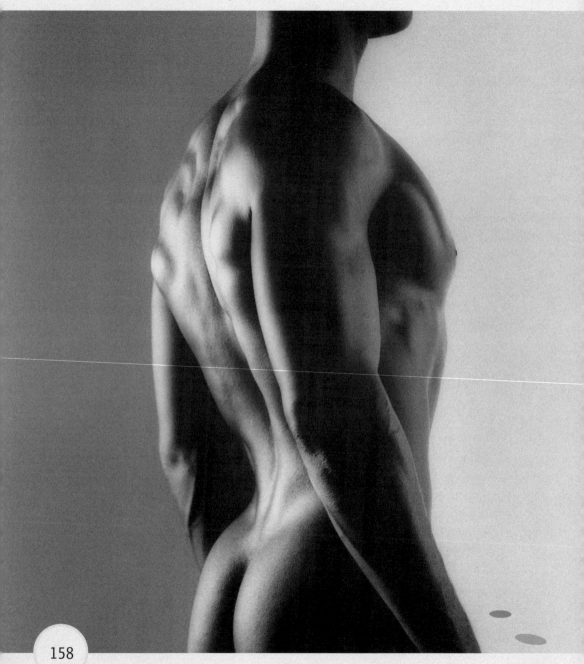

37

A little bit on the side

We all worry about what we look like from the front, and from the back, but rarely spend time thinking about our sides. When it comes to Pilates, however, a little bit on the side can be the perfect way to get long and strong.

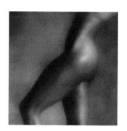

Think carefully about what Pilates exercises you do when left to your own devices and you'll probably find there's a pattern.

If you came to Pilates to correct a posture or back problem, then you'll probably still do the exercises prescribed for that. If, however, you came to it in order to slim and tone or to develop long, lean leg muscles, you've probably dropped the exercises you don't like by now and spend most of your mat time on your back with a few exercises focusing on your front. This is a very two-dimensional view of the body. Time to bring in the sides and work on that third dimension.

THE SIDE BEND

Stretch yourself out on the mat in a straight line on your left side. You can try and rest your feet side by side, one in front of the other, but if this means you are too unstable to control the movement properly, then slide one foot slightly back so that the edges of both feet are able to touch the floor and your ankles are slightly

Here's an idea for you...

In Joseph H.'s original version of the side bend you start on your right side, and breathe out and push yourself up onto one arm at arm's length from the floor, your body straight and your other arm straight down at your side. Inhaling slowly you turn your head to the left, chin to shoulder and lower the body until the right calf touches the floor while sliding the left hand down the thigh towards the knee. Exhale slowly and return to the straight position. Repeat three times only – this is more difficult because you are having to balance as you move which works the obliques more. As a variant Joseph recommended making life more interesting by having the left arm straight out above your head in line with your body.

crossed. Now scoop, park and breathe out as you lift yourself up on your left arm so you are at arm's length from the floor. Remember not to lock the elbow, and if this is too difficult a position to balance, then drop down so you are propped up on the elbow (which should be directly beneath your shoulder). Stretch the right arm up in the air and then drop it down over your head so you are as long as possible. Lift up the right hip (try pushing into the floor with the right foot) so that your spine has a little curve on it and think of yourself as a bow with one tip at your right foot, the other at your right hand, and try to stretch that bow out as long as possible. Relax back down and repeat with the other side. Three to six repetitions on each side should stretch your spine, serratus and obliques.

THE MERMAID

This is really a side bend with a slight twist. Start sitting on the floor with your legs bent and both tucked to the same side, let's say the left side in this case. Park the pelvis and scoop the stomach. Keep facing forward even though you'll now be resisting a twisting force from the position of your legs. Reach down and touch your left leg with your left hand or rest it on the floor. Raise your right arm up in the air above you and exhale as you bend that right side over towards your left. Inhale and return. Now smoothly raise your left arm and place your right hand on the ground beside you. Breathing out, bend your left arm over the top of your head. Imagine your hand is being pulled over your head and stretch the left hand side of your body as much as you can to let it move that way. Keep the neck long. Give it all the stretch you can, then breathe in again and return back to the centre. Rather than performing a multiple series of exercises you may want to give it your best in the one stretch on each side and leave it at that.

Side stretching can also be done while standing – take a look at IDEA 27, *Lateral thinking*.

Try another idea...

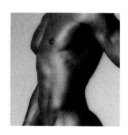

'Be free all worthy spirits, and stretch yourselves, for greatness and for height.'
GEORGE CHAPMAN, playwright

Defining idea...

161

How did
it go?

Q   **I like the feeling in my back as I perform the mermaid, but not the pain in my knee. Do I have to put up with that?**

A   *No, simply sit on a small cushion which will take the pressure off the knees. If that's not convenient, then try to stretch out the upper leg to one side and see if that helps.*

Q   **OK, so I agree that I want strong sides to my ribs and waist. How can I take moves like the mermaid and add strength work.**

A   *The mermaid lends itself very nicely to work on the Reformer if you want to add resistance to the stretching. See IDEA 36,* Rack and roll with the Reformer.

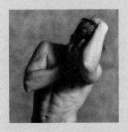

38

Wundaful

Don't be fooled by the name. There's nothing relaxing about chair work and the chances are you won't even get to sit down. What you will get, however, is a Wundaful workout.

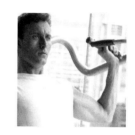

The big difference between the Wunda chair and the other machines described in this book is that many of the exercises performed on it are so different from their mat work equivalents as to be virtually unrecognisable.

Some instructors prefer to talk about Wunda chair exercises as an entirely different and specialised discipline. In general these exercises lean towards the more gymnastic and strength-oriented end of the spectrum.

The chair itself can come cunningly disguised in a number of ways. The original models are very simple to look at. They consist of a sturdy stool with a flat top and a platform or step projecting like a footrest. Take a closer look at that footrest and you'll see that it is spring loaded. Some manufacturers have added the further refinement of splitting that spring-loaded footrest into two rests to allow different

With the Reformer and the Cadillac it's possible to show how a familiar position like the Hundred is modified by the machine. The Wunda chair is a little more radical and you can't really adapt the Hundred to it in the same way. What you can do, however, is to break down elements of the Hundred's movements and work on them. So, for example, an instructor might have you work on Hundred footwork by having you perch on the seat top, hands gripping the side, and feet on the spring step which you push away as you breathe out and extend your legs. You might then work on your arms by squatting in front of the chair and performing the air-slap or pumping motion but with your hands resting on the spring step so that you have to push that down with each pumping movement to work the laterals and shoulders.

movements, and some models have sprouted handles and even chair backs – at which point the Wunda chair does actually start to look like a chair. (Well, it does if you get your ideas on furniture design from Salvador Dali.) Naturally enough most people assume that they will get to sit on the chair and probably put their feet on the rest. A reasonable enough assumption and there are positions where you do just that, although you're then expected to grip the seat top and push against the spring-loaded step as you extend the legs. A great many of the Wunda chair exercises, however, don't involve sitting down at all, and indeed you are just as likely to be asked to lie across the seat top on your back or side, to stand on the top, or to lie or kneel on the floor in front of it.

The trick to understanding the Wunda is not only to forget about the word 'chair' but also to stop seeing the springy platform as a step or footrest. It is just as often a bar for the arms to push against so that exercises include lying on the chair and straightening the arms, or squatting in front of the bar and pushing it down to the floor. You may be asked to stand on top and work one leg at a time, extending the hamstrings against the spring resistance. The hidden secret is that there is not one spring but four or five of different strengths so that the resistance can be raised or lowered as appropriate, depending on which muscles are being worked. After your first session you will also feel the stretch in your balancing and stabilising muscles. That's because a common feature of many exercises is that when you're perched on the chair pushing away at the bar you are also having to steady your core to avoid tipping off. It's harder than it looks, and it's great for that girdle of strength.

The Wunda chair may sound a bit daft (it's pronounced 'vunda' as in the German 'wunderbar') but it can offer a great alternative for when ordinary mat work seems a little stale and you feel like grappling (literally) with a new challenge.

Like contorting yourself around the chair and keen to explore the 'gymnastic' face of Pilates further? Then take a look at IDEA 40, *Roll out the barrel*, and find out about other pieces of equipment to cavort, curl and crunch with.

Try another idea...

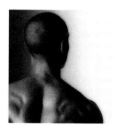

'There are many wonderful things, and nothing is more wonderful than man.'
SOPHOCLES

Defining idea...

Q **I was lying on my side and pushing the spring step away from me which felt fine until the next day when I stiffened up down my side. Why?**

A *That's the thing about the chair, it's harder than it looks because you are often concentrating on one movement while actually working another part of your body. In this case you felt the exercise was about your arm muscles because they were doing the visible work. In practice you were also balancing on your side and your obliques and serratus muscles of the ribcage were contracting to keep you in place and stabilise the movement. This is a good thing. Honest.*

Q **I tried it but it didn't do anything for me – it just felt easy pushing the spring back and forth. Am I missing something?**

A *Depends what you're trying to achieve. If you just get on and have a go you're unlikely to find it very useful. Try having a chat with your instructor about what you might gain from it. If you were trying it on an instructor's recommendation, tell them and maybe try something with more resistance, like the Reformer.*

39

Cruising in the Cadillac

It doesn't have wheels, it doesn't look like a car, in fact it looks like nothing more than a four-poster bed designed for the Marquis de Sade. Climb into the Cadillac.

If the Reformer is a post-apocalypse mutant rowing machine, then the Cadillac is very clearly the hardware of choice for the hardcore Pilates pervert.

Wrist straps dangle from a four-poster bed, ankle and thigh cuffs are often in evidence and as if any confirmation was needed some of these are fluffy with fake fur. If your Mum were to come across this piece of equipment in your house you'd have a lot of explaining to do.

Quite why it is called a Cadillac is a bit of a mystery. I was once assured that the name was a reference to the resistance springs and the comparison with the deep-sprung comfort of the car. This seems a little fanciful, and while I don't claim to be an expert in Cadillacs I doubt that many of their passengers travelled around strapped to the ceiling. Joseph H. used to call it a rehabilitation table, and its other common name is the trapeze table, either of which gives a much better idea of how it works and what it does.

Here's an idea for you... **While the most eye-catching images of the Caddy inevitably feature people suspended from the frame it may help understand the beast to consider an altogether more familiar pose. Just as the Reformer adds a new twist to the Hundred with resistance on the arms, so does the Cadillac, but with the added distinction that not only the amount of resistance, but the precise angle of pull can now be modified. Springs link the wrist cuffs to the top of the frame so that when performing the usual air-slaps with the hands those springs add resistance to the arm movements. So far, so like the Reformer. The difference is that there is a bar which runs across the top frame and that can be fixed at any point from one end to the other. Which means that the anchor point of those springs could be behind you, above you, down by your feet, or any point in between. Each variation subtly changes the angle of pull of the muscles and that can have implications for which muscles the body recruits to do the job. That fine degree of adjustment means a trained instructor can find out exactly how you are working your body and tweak the tasks so that you have to work in minutely different ways.**

If you take your eyes off the fluffy thigh cuffs for a minute you'd see that the Cadillac consists of a high table top set in the middle of a four-poster frame, which acts as a support for a series of springs and straps. The height of the table allows those with mobility problems to lie down easily, which gives the clue to the real nature of the beast. Unlike the Reformer, which is an exercise machine working by movement and resistance, the Cadillac is halfway between a piece of exercise equipment and an apparatus for physical therapy.

Where the Reformer works by moving yourself around by pulling or pushing on the sliding platform, the essence of Cadillac technique is more about static, often isometric exercise. In isometrics the muscles contract against something that doesn't move, rather than striving to lift a weight or fling a limb around. Originally designed as a piece of rehabilitation equipment for the bedridden, the Cadillac is designed to allow users to work on strength without having to take their own bodyweight. To do that the design incorporates a number of features including a 'trapeze', (picture the bar that trapeze artists hold on to), and a series of springs attached to bars that can be configured in a number of ways. These give the user different ways to get a grip on the caddy while lying on the tabletop or, more spectacularly, suspended from the frame using the aforementioned cuffs and loops. Because of the complexity of the Caddy you're unlikely to be encouraged to simply leap on and have a go. You really do need a qualified instructor to use it properly, but that doesn't mean it need be intimidating and although its principal purpose is treating those with injuries or problems it can also be a brilliant idea for solving tangled technique. If your studio has a caddy, don't hesitate to ask if it can be part of your Pilates tuition – you don't necessarily have to end up hanging from the bed-posts in order to benefit.

If the fluffy thigh cuffs don't turn you on because you prefer the idea of moving freely, uninhibited by loops and springs, but you still want to experiment with equipment to enhance your Pilates, then have a look at the Wunda chair in IDEA 38, *Wundaful*.

Try another idea...

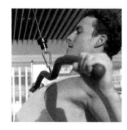

'Every boy's dream: a pink Cadillac.'
CLINT EASTWOOD, from the film *Pink Cadillac*

Defining idea...

How did it go?

Q **I'm a bit disappointed. Not only did I not get to be bound and dangled in exotic positions but more to the point my session seemed to consist of much the same exercises repeated over and over. Why?**

A *Some instructors forget that we want to know in detail what's going on, especially with new toys like the Caddy. The chances are that while you thought you were doing the same thing repeatedly the instructor was making fine changes to the Caddy's configuration to see how it affected your movements. What you need now is a thorough debrief. Try threatening to strap the instructor to the Caddy unless he explains just what it is he has learnt.*

Q **I liked it but found it too easy. How can I make it tougher?**

A *You sure you want to? If you're using the Cadillac it's usually as therapy for a problem and you should let the instructor guide you on degrees of toughness. If, however, you're sure you want more resistance, then ask the instructor to reset the springs to make it harder to do the same moves.*

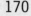

40

Roll out the barrel

Watch someone working the barrel and you'll instantly see the link between Pilates and the world of dance. Fortunately you don't have to be a Fonteyn, Nureyev or Billy Elliot to make it as a barrelina.

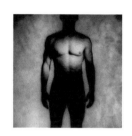

Barrels are the Pilates equivalent of the ballet bar you see in front of the mirrors in dance studios.

But where ballet bars are mainly for balance as you plié or to put the foot up on, the whole-body approach of Pilates means that barrelinas are expected to twist and turn pretty much every part of themselves around the barrel to get that extra stretch. There are several types of barrels but they are all props to help position the body so that you can get a concentrated, controlled stretch, usually in the legs and hips. If the Wunda chair (see IDEA 38, *Wundaful*) appeals to the more gymnastic end of the Pilates spectrum, the barrels undoubtedly attract the dancers. That doesn't mean you have to don a tutu to use one (though no one's going to stop you if that's your thing) and the barrels are just as helpful for runners or roofers.

LADDER BARREL

Just what it says on the box. A rounded surface like a large barrel is fixed to a plinth which also has a short ladder of rungs rising up from the floor. The plinth is actually

Here's an idea for you...

Start by sitting on the ladder barrel facing the ladder and with your feet secured by tucking them under the rungs. Now breathe in and arch gently back over the barrel so that your spine curls backwards following the barrel's curve. Now breathe out and perform the curl up, using your abdominals to lift your body back up to the sitting position. This is a tough exercise and will really work you hard, but it combines with a very satisfying back stretch at the bottom of the move. Make sure you come up smoothly, not jerkily, and resist the temptation to move your arms as counterbalances to try and help pull you up. If you're really confident you have good form and a tungsten tum, then fold your arms across your chest throughout the exercise. Complete three to six repetitions, then turn over and lie across the barrel face down to feel the stretch in your spine the other way.

a sliding base that means the difference between ladder and barrel can be adjusted to allow for anyone from petite ballerina to brick-outhouse-sized builders.

Perhaps the simplest way of using the ladder barrel is to take hold of the top rung of the ladder and treat it like the ballet bar in a dance studio – with the difference that you have the barrel to put your leg up on to. Hamstring, hip and thigh stretches like these need some practice before you launch your limbs at the top of a high barrel, and even for the experienced they shouldn't be attempted without warming the muscle first to increase its elasticity.

Hip and ham stretches are only the tip of the iceberg of the barrel's repertoire. The curving top to the barrel is designed so that you can curve your spine over it safely, achieving a deep arch with support (see Here's an idea for you for more).

ARC BARREL

Ladder barrels are a barrel of laughs but they are big and bulky and don't really lend themselves to group sessions. Enter the arc barrel. These are lightweight, portable half barrels covered with comfy upholstering to help support your back or shoulders. The idea is much like the use of the Swiss ball in back stretches, but without the instability of the ball. This makes the arc barrels much more suitable for those recovering from injury or tenderly trying to untwist the kinks of a bad back. That said, the smaller barrels are also becoming increasingly popular in group sessions to spice up mat work and enable deeper stretches. Some half barrels also have handholds cut into the sides to help you get a grip when draping yourself over them.

Try another idea...

Supported stretching is a great feeling but you don't have to have access to barrels to do it. Take a look at stretching on the Swiss ball in IDEA 29, *On the ball I*.

SPINE CORRECTOR AND SPINE SUPPORTER

You may also come across the name spine corrector used for the arc barrel, and there is a variant called the step barrel (not to be confused with the ladder barrel) which is really an arc barrel combined with an angled step/seat. The spine supporter, on the other hand, is a half-moon shape designed to slip under the spine as you work and aimed at those who are prevented from doing some mat work exercises due to a weak lower back. It's also particularly popular among pregnant Pilates practitioners.

Defining idea...

'Roll out the barrel, we'll have a barrel of fun
Roll out the barrel, we've got the blues on the run.'
Popular refrain for drinking/dynamic stretching

Q **I am using the ladder barrel to help me with my classic leg raise stretches but what can it help me do that I can't do with a ballet bar?**

A *You may be letting your ballet bar experience shape your movements on the barrel. Dancers often approach a bar and stand side on out of habit. Try standing facing the ladder and with the barrel behind you. You can now bend your knee and place your foot on the barrel to stretch the quads, or use the barrel to support your leg stretched out behind you.*

Q **I'm very tall and so putting my leg up on the barrel for a stretch is too easy. How can I use it then?**

A *Tallness is no problem. For the classic hamstring stretch place one leg on the top of the barrel (easy since you are so tall) and then slowly bend the standing leg so that you 'sit' down into the stretch and your resting leg is stretched. That should also work your glutes (bum) and thighs.*

41

Feelin' good

Every Pilates move is designed to help with balance, poise and strength, but some of them are worth it anyway just because they feel so good. Here are a couple of moves to help you soothe jangled nerves or reward yourself for a hard morning.

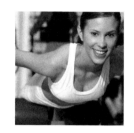

Yes, Pilates is about strengthening, toning and balancing and, yes, Pilates can bring all of that into your daily life as you go about working, exercising, shopping, travelling and simply sitting down.

Pilates is immensely energising – it's the only exercise I know where I can leave an hour-long group class and feel fresher than when I went in – but sometimes you just want to take a break. So here are some ideas for moves and positions which are unashamedly all about simply feeling good.

CAT STRETCH

This is a great little stretch to wake up those back muscles and in particular the erector spinae that run the length of your backbone and bend it backwards.

If all this is making you feel so good you actually want to add a bit of work to it, then you can beef up the hip rolls to tone the obliques more and work towards your wafer-thin waistline.

Assume the position for the normal hip roll but this time bend your knees at right angles and instead of resting your feet on the floor hold them up in the air so that your calves are parallel to the floor. This time you're not going to relax as you place your knees down to the side but instead focus on the movement. Breathe out as you move the legs over to one side and your head to the other. If you can't twist far enough to place the knees on the ground, don't worry about it, just lower them as far towards the floor as is comfortable and then breathe in again for another five-second count and gently sway the bent legs over the other way while rolling your neck in the opposite direction.

Start on all fours, your hands shoulder-width apart directly beneath the shoulders, and fingers spread. Remember not to lock you elbows and make sure you scoop the stomach and park the pelvis. Now breathe out and arch the spine right up, tucking your chin down towards your chest and pushing upwards right through the middle of your shoulder blades to open out your chest. Hold it for a moment, and then breathe in and slowly lower back to the starting point. Repeat for, well, as many repetitions as you fancy actually.

RESTING CHILD

Having started with the cat stretch it's great to go straight into the 'resting child', not least because you're already on your hands and knees.

Bring your feet together and lower your bum so that you're sitting on them. At the same time bend your elbows so that you lower yourself down until your forearms are flat on the floor. You should now look much like a Muslim at prayer. In purist Pilates thinking this is now the moment to practice your back breathing. Some people like to have a small towel at hand to prop under their forehead if they're planning on staying some time in this position. That's particularly handy if you want to try this yoga variant on the 'resting child'; rest your forehead on the mat/towel and gently pull your arms back behind you, resting them

Stretching hitting the spot? Try taking it to the next level with stretching over a Swiss ball – read IDEA 29, *On the ball I.*

Try another idea…

alongside you on the floor with the palms upwards and next to your feet. Both versions of 'resting child' are supremely relaxing but some people prefer the yoga variant because of the way it drops their shoulders. Breathe deeply and easily and try not to think about the rent/report/row that's been winding you up. Switch from the cat to the child as often as you need to feel good.

HIP ROLLS

This is meant to be a mobility exercise and does lightly work the oblique muscles at the sides of your torso but I tend to do it just to unwind. Lie flat on your back and take the time to think about your spinal alignment and neutral pelvis. Slide your shoulders down your spine and think about where your back is making contact with the floor. Your knees should be bent with your feet flat on the floor. Now spread your arms out to each side, scoop that stomach and breathe out for a five-second count as you roll your head in one direction and your bent knees in the other so that that they rest (still bent) on top of each other, the lower one on the ground. Relax and sink into the stretch for as long as you want, then breathe out again and switch sides so the head turns the other way and the legs go to the opposite side.

'*Watch a cat as it lazily opens its eyes, slowly looks around, and gradually prepares to rise after a nap. First it gradually rises on its hindquarters and then gradually lowers itself again, at the same time sprawling out on the floor, leisurely stretching its forepaws and legs.*'
JOSEPH H. PILATES

Defining idea…

177

Q **I love the combination of the cat and child and the stretch it gives the length of my back, but can I take it any further by sitting on the floor rather than on my heels?**

A *Best not. It's not considered the best position for the spine. Instead, if you want to extend the stretch, keep your ankles together so you're still sitting on your heels but open the knees a bit further apart and try to sink your chest down between them. That should give you a stretch down your inner thigh.*

Q **In the hip roll does it matter how tightly my knees are in to my chest?**

A *It affects the muscles used. If you have tight hip flexors you may feel uncomfortable pulling your knees right up, but be careful because the further away from your chest your knees are the more work your obliques will perform to complete the move.*

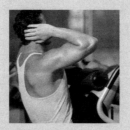

42

Shake a leg

**Striving for strength but not wild about weights? Try a
different kind of weight, then, and shake a leg.**

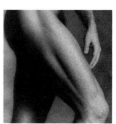

Ankle weights are definitely back in
fashion. Once only the very hardcore or
mildly masochistic could be seen sporting them
but now the leading sport fashion companies are
selling them and they've even put in an
appearance in the Pilates studio.

It's not too hard to understand why. For a start people are often quite happy about
the idea of adding weights to their workout, but put off by clutching at dumbbells.
Then there's the problem of how to add weight to the smaller leg exercises (you
ever tried to clutch a dumbbell with your toes?). In addition, the benefits of weights
work in overcoming osteoporosis are becoming better known and so there is a
move towards getting heavy – but without dumbbelling down. Ankle weights are
the answer to all of those issues. They are bright and comfortable, with the wonder
that is velcro making them easy to slip on and off and adjust to size. They come in a
variety of sizes and weights and it's no longer social death to be seen with them in
public.

Here's an idea for you...

Ankle weights don't just fit on ankles. They're also great on wrists too. Work on the Reformer (see IDEA 36, *Rack and roll with the Reformer*) shows how adding resistance can beef up almost any Pilates move, and wrist weights can be used to add resistance to any hand gesture from the Hundred to the seated twist.

ABDUCTOR AND ADDUCTOR EXERCISES

The abductors are the muscles around the top of the thighs and hips that open the legs, the adductors are the muscles of the inner thigh that close them. Together they give a toned look to the top of the leg and strengthening them will help avoid injuries, particularly those from suddenly changing direction (footballers take note). As with most paired muscles you should make sure that if you work one, you work the other. Otherwise you risk strengthening one at the expense of the other and such imbalances can affect posture.

First lie on your right side, making sure your spine is in line and resting your head on your right arm. Lightly bend your right leg at the knee for stability and scoop the stomach. Straighten your left leg and turn the whole leg in slightly from the hip so that the ankle is uppermost. Now breathe out as you raise the leg 15–20 cm (6–8 inches) off the ground and breathe back in as you lower. Ten repetitions on each side.

For the adductor exercises it may help to have a chair handy. Lie on your right side as before but this time resting your left leg on a chair seat and with your right leg straight (remembering not to lock the knee). Because you don't have a bent knee underneath you for support, you may want to extend your left hand out forwards to the ground in front of your chest. Breathe out and lift your right leg as if to meet your left leg. When it touches the bottom of the chair seat (that your left leg is resting on) hold for a moment, then breathe in and return to the start position. Ten repetitions again on each side.

HAMSTRING

The hamstring is the muscle at the back of the thigh that bends the knee. The standard Pilates move to isolate it is the one leg kick. Lie face down with your legs out straight behind you. You may find it more comfortable to raise your chest and rest on your elbows, but if so be careful not to arch your back – keep your shoulders low as this is not the 'full cobra' (see IDEA 34, *Yogalates*).

Breathe out and bend your left knee, raising the ankle towards the buttock. Joseph H. used to recommend 'snap-kicking' for this but these days there are plenty of other people ready to kick your arse without doing it yourself, so the approved approach now is to take it nice and steady. Breathe in and return. Swap legs and repeat for ten repetitions on each side. One variation Joe did recommend was keeping the non-lifting leg straight but slightly off the ground throughout the move so as to work the erector spinae muscles.

There is almost no limit to the use of ankle weights. They can add resistance to everything from stretches to the more dynamic activities such as the kneeling side kick shown in IDEA 22, *Take that!* Just remember, though, that they do change the balance of your body and so exercises such as rolling (IDEA 25, *Foetal attraction*) will suddenly become very much more tricky.

Try another idea...

Another great way of adding resistance without resorting to pumping iron is to try a resistance band – see IDEA 32, *Your flexible friend II*.

Defining idea...

'I have two doctors – my left leg and my right leg.'
G. M. TREVELYAN, historian

How did it go?

Q   Should this be making my ankles tired?

A   Definitely not, no. Make sure of two things: the first is that your ankle should not be loose so that your foot flops around like a dying fish. The second is that you should not turn your foot at the ankle at all, but instead turn it inwards like a dancer from the hip so the whole leg pivots and your heel ends up higher than the ball of your foot.

Q   If ankle/wrist weights add punch to Pilates poses, what about those weight vests I see on sale next to them?

A   It's true that adding weight around your torso will make balancing muscles work harder, so if you fancy it, then why not? A word of warning: if you run or jump with a weight vest you'll be adding a lot of unexpected stress to your joints, particularly your knees.

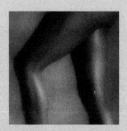

43

So hip it hurts

Your psoas or hip flexors are crucial to our entire posture, but most of us don't know where they are or what they do until something goes wrong.

Be honest, had you ever heard of your psoas muscles before? Even if we call them hip flexors could you explain where they start and end?

What they join to what? Would it surprise you to know that they not only affect how you move but will shape the way that you stand, and if too tight will cause a condition called lordosis or 'hollow back'? Read on and find out how to soften up your psoas and keep your hip flexors flexy.

I remember how I first learnt about hip flexors. Some time back I took up running to try and put some life back in an otherwise pretty clapped-out body. I loved the fresh air, I found it oddly therapeutic, and while my calves and thighs obviously got tired (usually before I made it past the newsagent on the corner) that was just fine because, well, I was running – what did I expect? What I definitely didn't expect was a bizarre ache in the top of my thighs, a very deep ache that seemed to reach right into the core of my wobbly being. As I hobbled stiff-legged into the physio's

Here's an idea for you...

If you're confident that your psoas are lithe, lissom and lovely, then try 'the teaser' to work those suckers some more. The teaser starts off on your back with your knees bent and arms straight up above your head on the floor. Straighten one leg up into the air and then breathe out and extend your hands out like a sleepwalker while rolling your spine off the floor one vertebra at a time. Breathe in and straighten your back at the high point of the lift (your hands should be up reaching for your toes) and then breathe out as you lower yourself back down one vertebra at a time.

office he had already uttered the words 'hip flexors' seemingly before even looking up. I've taken great care of them ever since.

One of the reasons why it dwells in obscurity is that you can't see your psoas. The psoas muscle is what brings the knee up to the chest (or vice versa), and it runs from the lower spine right through the pelvic girdle and attaches to the thigh bone. If it isn't worked and stretched it can become tight, and that means a couple of things. The first is that the day you are late for that plane and bound up the stairs to the departure lounge it will resent you bitterly and leave you feeling like you've pulled something. The second is that it will exert undue pressure on the spine itself, tugging the lower spine forwards and causing the small of the back to become more exaggerated. If you spend all day sat down (in which position the psoas are shortened) and use lifts and elevators rather than stairs you increase the chances of tight psoas.

We all have a certain amount of curvature of the spine, but if you lie flat on the floor and find that you can't straighten out your legs without arching your back, then your psoas is probably tight. Normally the psoas is countered by abdominal muscles, but if they too have become less than steely, then we have a recipe for lower back trouble. Because the psoas affects both spinal alignment and core strength it is very close to the heart (OK, the groin) of Pilates practitioners.

Footballers limber up their psoas by slow running in which you pull your knees up as high as they can go with a movement like a trotting horse. That's all very well for them but the rest of us risk groin injury if we aren't used to that and would be well advised to concentrate on gentle stretching before launching into hip flexion frenzy.

Fancy swinging those psoas around? Well if you're confident they're strong enough, take a look at the kneeling side kick in IDEA 22, Take that!

Try another idea...

YOU FLEXY BEAST

Lie flat on your back with both legs bent and your feet flat on the floor. Scoop the stomach and park the pelvis as ever, and then breathe in and bring your left knee up to your chest and hold the knee in both hands. Now breathe out and extend the right leg out along the floor as long as you can. It's very important at this point to focus on your spine and pelvis rather than on the bent leg or the leg doing the moving. You should be feeling for any attempt by your back to realign itself instead of letting the psoas muscles stretch out. Breathe in and slide the right leg back up to the start, breathe out and gently lower the left leg back down to its starting point.

'I got kicked out of ballet class because I pulled a groin muscle. It wasn't mine.'
RITA RUDNER, American comedian, illustrating just one of the dangers of getting gung-ho with groins

Defining idea...

How did
it go?

Q   I tried the flexy beast stretch and can feel it in my hip flexors, but how do I know I'm getting it right?

A   As you perform the stretch feel carefully for what's going on in your lower back. If you feel any arching as you extend the leg on the ground, then repeat the stretch until you can do it without the back arching at all.

Q   I tried the teaser and it's not my hip flexors that suffer, it's my lower stomach. Is that right?

A   Yes it is. Keeping the weight of your legs off the floor is the job of the lower abdominals so they will be doing the work.

44

Bending over backwards

In the car, at the keyboard and of course slaving over a hot stove – we spend most of our lives bent over forwards. Time to redress the balance a little and bend over backwards to please yourself, for once.

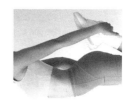

When future social historians get to have a few chuckles over our lives and times I suspect that one of the ones that will crease them up is just how much time we spend creased up.

We spend half our lives sitting down – at desks, at tables, or in cars – and since most of us are too tired to take proper care of posture we're effectively slumped forwards, sagging gently at the waist. Then because those waists start to do a bit of gentle sagging of their own, we high-tail it down to the nearest gym and try to look a little bit more like our big-screen idols. Which usually means doing sit-ups or crunches. Great, more bending over, just what we needed. The irony is that while a gut can give you back trouble by pulling you out balance, many of us try to sort that out by strengthening our six-pack. But if the six-pack isn't balanced by the back muscles that can only make matters worse. The madness of modern life isn't showing any

Here's an idea for you...

You can take the swan dive a step further by removing your triceps from the equation so that the whole movement is performed by alternating contractions of your back muscles and abdominals. Start off just as for the normal swan dive, but when you straighten your arms and rise up to the top of the movement, take your hands off the floor and stick them out straight ahead of you like Superman in full flight. This should make you start to rock forwards and you should continue to rock as far forward up your chest as you can with you legs rising as high off the floor as is comfortable before rocking backwards. Continue to rock backwards and forwards for three to five movements of each.

For the full Joseph H. version of this move, don't hold your arms forwards in Superman pose, but instead throw them out sideways and slightly backwards. If you think about it you will now look like an Acapulco cliff diver (in this case one with a severe fear of heights) and the name of this exercise will suddenly become clear to you.

signs of abating, so let's try and do a little bit to even things up by flexing our spines the other way – literally bending over backwards.

DOUBLE HEEL KICKS

You might be surprised that this and the other exercises take place lying on your front. It really is the safest way to bend over backwards. Lie on your front on the mat and turn your head to one side (because breathing is so much nicer than sucking mat) and put your arms behind your back, one hand in the other. Scoop that stomach and park that pelvis in neutral. Breathe out and quickly kick both feet up towards your buttocks three times. Breathe in and stretch the legs back straight out and as high up off the floor as you feel comfortable with. Squeeze your shoulders together and push your arms back as far as you can towards your feet.

This will bring your chest up off the floor, breathe in as you lift your head and chest and extend the neck up to open the chest and back. Breathe out again and return your body to the starting position. Repeat for a total of ten repetitions.

SWAN DIVE

Another great backwards bending exercise, but one to approach with some caution. If you're not used to swan diving (also known as the rocking press-up), then warm up to it gently with normal back raises.

For the sake of balance you may want to combine these bending over backwards exercises with their equal and opposite counterparts. Turn to IDEA 25, *Foetal attraction*, to find out about rolling up forwards like a ball.

Try another idea...

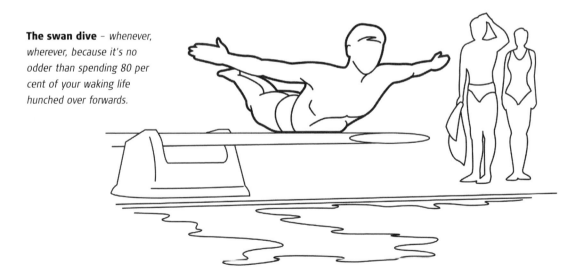

The swan dive – *whenever, wherever, because it's no odder than spending 80 per cent of your waking life hunched over forwards.*

'I bend and do not break.'
JEAN DE LA FONTAINE

The starting point for the swan dive is rather like a collapsed press-up. Lie on your stomach on the mat with your hands in the press-up position, shoulder-width apart. Scoop the stomach and raise the legs off the ground. Breathe out and straighten your arms, pushing your chest off the mat and lifting your head up. Once at the top of the movement breathe in and bend the arms to rock your body forwards so that the legs rise in the air as high as you can comfortably manage. Breathe out again and straighten the arms to rock back. The whole move should be fluid and continuous, not jerky. This is about control as well as strengthening your backbone.

How did it go?

Q I tried the double heel kick but get real tension in my shoulders. How do I avoid that?

A *Remember to squeeze the shoulder blades down the back as much as you can and extend the neck out as if growing it. You may also want to reduce the intensity of your bending backwards until your body adjusts.*

Q I've tried the swan dive and I just can't bend backwards enough to complete it. How do I improve?

A *Simply practice the press-up position but keep your legs on the floor throughout the move. Concentrate on lifting up your chest as much as you can and bending the spine backwards. This will develop the flexibility and strength that you can later convert into the full body arc needed to complete the swan dive.*

45

Secrets of the Magic Circle

Joseph Pilates' Magic Circle has been doing the rounds for decades. Find out why you're never to old to play with a ring-pull.

If you thought Pilates was all about lissom-limbed loveliness and 'Sex and the City'-style sophistication you might reasonably wonder what on earth a giant ring-pull has to do with it at all.

Having learnt from the cock up of 'Contrology' (the name never stuck), Joseph Pilates had clearly got his head around the idea of marketing by the time he came to invent the Magic Circle. It's a very fancy name indeed for what is, after all, a simple circle of steel or plastic. As with everything else to do with Pilates it has since been seized on by ever more modern marketers and repackaged as, among others, the Fitness Circle, the Spring Circle, the Power Circle, and in a blatant bid to out-circle the other circles the awesome-sounding Ultra-Fit Circle. My own favourite is the Flex Ring Toner, but the less said about that the better.

No matter which of the many brands you end up with in your hands, your own first reaction will inevitably be 'Oh…'. The names may be grand but in the end what you get is a stiff but flexible circle with a cushioned pad on each side – not really very

One of the favourite uses for a Magic Circle is to help with adductor work on the inner thigh. Lying on your back, trap the circle between the insides of your knees so that each knee is resting on the cushioned pads. Scoop the stomach, park the pelvis and breathe out for a slow five count as you push the knees together and compress the circle. Breathe in as you slowly release and return to the start position.

inspiring at first sight. In practice, however, the circle is an appropriately well-rounded performer.

The circles can be put to use in combination with any number of mat work exercises, whether standing, sitting or lying down. The basic moves consist of either compressing the circle or pulling against it as a resistance band. Working with it as a resistance band might mean looping the circle over the foot of an outstretched leg and pulling back the ball of the foot to get a better hamstring stretch. Compressing it could mean holding the pads on either side in the hands in front of the chest and simply trying to push the hands together to work the pectorals. Although there is a degree of movement, this kind of exercise is edging towards the field of isometrics where muscles are worked by contracting them against something that moves little if at all. Contrast with a dumbbell exercise, where the resistance moves a great deal, and you'll see that the fixed resistance of the ring isn't so good for working a muscle through its full range of movement. The flip side is that when compressing a circle you are expected to hold it against the resistance and it's at that point you realise how tough these frail looking objects really are.

Depending on how flexible or how resistant they are, different circles lend themselves better to pulling or compressing.

Some circles are designed to be high resistance and tough to compress. One model is steel, weighs in at 1 kg, and bears comparison with a chest expander. If you're too young or too sophisticated to know what a chest expander was, it consisted of a number of springs with a handle at each end. Would-be Charles Atlases (the Arnie of his day) would pose for hours in front of the bedroom mirror, trying very hard

If you're looking for resistance work you can do at home and you're not wild about weights, then take a look at resistance bands, which are cheap, easy to use and extremely portable. For more, turn to IDEA 31, *Your flexible friend I*.

Try another idea...

to pull the springs open across their chests. Great care had to be taken in case you reached muscle failure or your hand slipped, at which point the springs would contract violently with potentially dire consequences for the nipples. It was with a nostalgic sigh that I read of one reviewer who suffered the modern day equivalent when a steel sprung circle made a bolt for it while being squeezed between his knees. Male readers are already crossing their legs at the thought of what happens when a high-tensile steel spring is released between the thighs.

In a studio you're most likely to come across the lighter, more flexible plastic circles. If you like using the circle, this is also a good type to buy: you can throw it into an overnight bag and not notice it's there when it's time to take your Pilates on the road.

'Magic is believing in yourself, if you can do that, you can make anything happen.'
JOHANN WOLFGANG VON GOETHE

Defining idea...

How did it go?

Q Can the circle be used for anything other than resistance work?

A *Yes. Circles can also be used as a concentration tool and some teachers like to employ them for exercises like the teaser (see IDEA 43, So hip it hurts). The idea is that in exercises where both feet are off the ground, you hold the circle between the ankles. The co-ordination of doing that and the concentration of mind and muscle results in a much deeper workout for the stabilising and core muscles.*

Q My studio has very light flexible circles. How would I use these for resistance work?

A *More flexible circles are mainly used to pull against, much like a large rubber band, and so they can be looped around both feet, for example, with the effort being to try and pull the feet apart.*

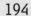

46

Backbones and bolsters

Bolstering your backbone is as easy as falling off a white plastic log with the foam roller.

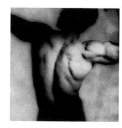

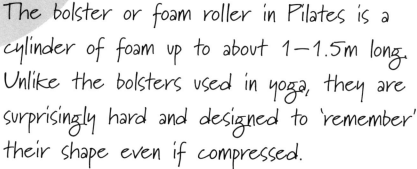

The bolster or foam roller in Pilates is a cylinder of foam up to about 1–1.5m long. Unlike the bolsters used in yoga, they are surprisingly hard and designed to 'remember' their shape even if compressed.

They've been used for a long time in physiotherapy where it's common to rest your bodyweight on the roller and then roll it over the affected area (thigh, hamstring, etc.). The Pilates foam roller is often said to have originated as a prop for the Feldenkrais method (see IDEA 28, *What the Feldenkrais!?*). In Pilates they are rarely used as rollers, but are usually lain on lengthways, resting the length of your spine along the roller. That stretches the chest, straightens the spine and helps with the postural muscles. It also opens up the ribcage to help with breathing exercises. Increasingly popular in group classes, they are cheap and so easy to buy for the home but they don't compress so they do tend to take up a lot of space.

You can also use the roller as an instability device. To bring in the instability all you have to do is lift your feet up. Not both at once of course: that would have you unceremoniously dumped off the roller in a jiffy. No, instead you need to lift up just one leg at a time. Keep the knee bent at 90 degrees and breathe out for a count of five seconds as you lift one knee up towards your chest. This is a good stretch for the hip flexors but most of all for the abdominals, including the obliques, as they are forced to stabilise not only the roll of the roller, but the fact that your pelvis will tip after a certain point in the lift and that will change your spinal alignment and thus your balance. Breathe in again as you lower the leg, change legs and repeat for three to five repetitions on each side.

Defining idea...

'The equilibrium you admire in me is an unstable one, difficult to maintain.'
LEOPOLD SENGHOR, Senegalese poet and statesman

CHEST STRETCH

Lay the foam roller on the mat and sit down at one end of the cylinder, then roll down, one vertebra at a time, until you are lying full-length on it. If that's hard to do, and remember the roller will try and roll to one side or the other underneath you, then put your hands on the floor to steady yourself rather than risk slipping off. The roller should fit in between your shoulder blades and your spine should align with it. Keep your knees bent and your feet flat on the floor for stability. Don't be fooled by its white foam disguise – the roller is nothing more than a white plastic log and as we all know there is nothing easier than falling off a log. This is one time when you don't have to worry so much about parking in neutral because the instability of the roller means that the main thing here is just staying on top of it. Breathe out and stretch your arms straight up in the air, then breathe in and slowly let the shoulder blades sink down as far as they can on each side of the roller. That should put a stretch right into your ribcage and right across the pectoral muscles of the chest.

CURL-UPS

Now try curl-ups on the roller. From the lying position, tip the chin towards the chest and curl up the spine one vertebra at a time. You can really feel the spine on the roller as you do this and the instability of the roller means that your abs will not only be working to curl you up but also to keep on top of the lateral movement. If you want to add another layer of complexity to what is otherwise a very simple move, you can also lodge a small ball between your knees (see IDEA 47, *Small balls*) which will engage the adductor muscles of the inside of the thigh and in turn activate the deeper abdominals along with the six-pack.

To compare and contrast the different ways of bringing instability to the party turn to IDEA 24, *Balls to the wall*, and see how the ball can be used to support the back in a very different way while engaging the stabilising muscles.

Try another idea...

Q Why does it hurt?

How did it go?

A   If it hurts to lie on the bolster, then you're probably not ready for it yet. Some people find it quite uncomfortable just to lie on because it's a hard surface, but if it hurts as you move around, then you should go back to doing the exercises on the mat alone.

Q Feels good – is there any way to make the chest stretch deeper?

A   Yes. There is a variation in which instead of having your arms straight up, you put them straight out behind your head with the palms up. Then bend the elbows and slide the shoulder blades down the spine while lowering the elbow to the floor.

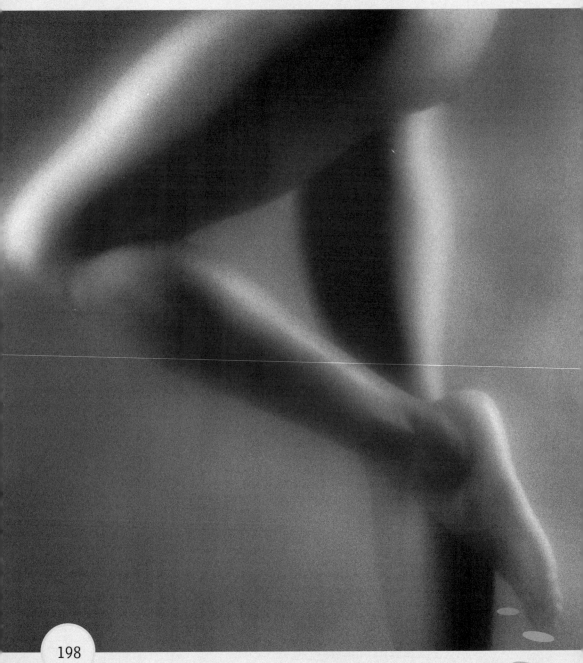

47

Small balls

Good things do come in small packages. Small balls punch above their weight by activating those hard to get at deep abs.

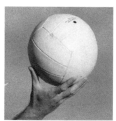

If you haven't worked out with Swiss balls then you haven't lived, but size really isn't everything — their baby brothers can play an equally important part in perfecting your Pilates technique.

Where the Swiss balls are mainly used to take all or some of the bodyweight and provide support, the small ball is used as a focus aid, a means of concentrating both the mind and the relevant muscle on the job in hand.

Just how small is a small ball depends on you – for some the small ball means something the size of a football, for others it can be as small as a tennis ball. Experiment and find what pleases you best. One thing though: it mustn't be heavy or hard to hold, so leather footballs and the like are out, not least since they tend to slip away when gripped between the knees.

Here's an idea for you... **If you enjoy the challenge of keeping a small ball in place as you work, then try the corkscrew with a small ball. The corkscrew is much like the jackknife featured in IDEA 52, *Topsy turvy II*, and starts from exactly the same position. Lying on your back, take your legs up and over so your body is on the shoulders and upper arms as in the shoulder stand (IDEA 51, *Topsy turvy I*). Instead of snapping your legs to the vertical as you do for the jackknife, twist your trunk to one side and lower both legs together towards the floor and back in a circular movement. The movement is then repeated on the other side. Remember that this time you have a small ball between your ankles: try very hard not to drop it. This is more difficult than with the roll over because as the legs go down to the side they slide over each other and the one nearest the floor ends up 'longer'. That's usually when I drop the ball.**

The thinking behind using a small ball gripped between the knees is that it makes you work the adductor muscles of the inner thigh and these are linked to the deeper abdominals and in particular the transversus. Force one to work, goes the theory, and you'll automatically lead the other to kick in. Try even a simple abs exercise holding the ball between your knees and you'll feel the difference. Here are a few ideas for using the ball to activate your abs.

CURL-UP WITH SMALL BALL

Pilates doesn't include crunches or sit-ups and instead has its own basic abs move – the curl-up. A curl-up is much smoother than a crunch and focuses on the Pilates trademark of rolling the spine up like a wheel, one vertebra at a time. Here we perform a normal curl-up but with the ball.

Lie on your back with your knees bent, feet flat on the ground and with a small ball lodged between your knees. Press the knees together, seeking to tense the inner thighs, scoop the stomach, park the pelvis, drop the chin towards the chest and breathe out for a count of five as you start to roll the spine up one vertebra at a time. Rise up as high as you are comfortable with, and then curl back just as slowly.

ROLL OVER WITH SMALL BALL

This is a touch trickier so you may need to experiment before finding the size of small ball that suits you best. Personally I lose more tennis balls this way...

For more exercises where you could use a small ball to add to the fun, take a look at IDEA 20, *Hundreds and thousands*. As well as the ball balanced on your belly, you can use one gripped between your knees to activate the adductors.

Try another idea...

Take a look at the roll over (IDEA 50, *Backtastic II*) and assume the same position but with the addition of a small ball gripped between the legs at the ankles.

On the back with the arms down by your sides and palms down slide your shoulder blades down the back, scoop the stomach, park the pelvis, and lift the legs up to the vertical. Roll the legs over the top to bring the toes down towards the floor above your head. Remember never to roll up onto your neck but instead stop at the shoulders. Try not to lose the ball (this is another exercise where a ball boy wouldn't be out of place). It's harder to get the same tension in the adductor muscles this way, but that's made up for by the muscle control required to keep that ball in place.

'Happiness is a ball after which we run wherever it rolls, and we push it with our feet when it stops,'
JOHANN WOLFGANG VON GOETHE

Defining idea...

How did
it go?

Q **I keep losing the ball in the roll over and corkscrew. What am I doing wrong?**

A *It's most likely that you don't quite have the full control as you perform the move (the ball is very unforgiving like that). Try breaking the moves down to their simplest forms like the ordinary roll over and the shoulder stand and make sure you've mastered the components before you put them all together with the ball.*

Q **Can I use a ball in any exercise?**

A *Pretty much any exercise where your feet or knees are together and off the floor yes. A tennis ball gripped at knee or ankle may help you concentrate on everything from the Hundred to the crunch.*

48

Forearm smash

If you've read IDEA 7, *Workhorses and whippets*, you'll know that part of the Pilates philosophy is to put mind and body in balance by favouring some of the smaller muscles rather than the workhorses that otherwise take over any given job.

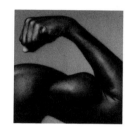

With the legs this means remembering to take the time to tone the muscles of the feet and shin as much as the thighs and buttocks. With the arms it means remembering that our arm muscles don't stop at the elbow.

Men and women alike will work to tone triceps and build biceps but very rarely do any exercises for the forearms, wrists and fingers. IDEA 11, *Pilates at the keyboard*, showed you how to stretch those parts of your body, now let's look at ways of building their strength.

When it comes to muscle celebrity the biceps are right up there at the top of the A-list, and while the triceps don't get so many starring roles they still get invited to all the good parties. Meanwhile the poor old flexor and extensor carpi ulnaris are stuck

Some people like to use a roller to strengthen their hands and wrists and find something oddly therapeutic about the action. You can make a simple wrist roller with nothing more complex than a short rod or handle, a bit of string and a weight. Tie the string to the weight at one end, and the middle of the rod at the other. The exercise consists of holding the rod with both hands palm down, as if you were about to be pulled off on water skis (another act of wrist-strengthening perhaps?), and turning it in both hands so the string wraps around the rod and lifts the weight. When the weight gets to the top you simply reverse the direction and start to lower it again. The art is to get the weight right for your strength: a little experimentation with likely objects should see you right.

in the kitchen doing the dishes along with the brachoradialis. Any reference to exercising the poor old flexor carpi radialis (the wrist flexor) usually raises nothing more than a snigger. Face it, nobody knows what the muscles of the forearm are and we rarely bother to isolate them and work on them. Yet the wrist flexors add power to so many things we do – and many sports demand strength and control at the wrist. Well, this is where you get to put things to rights, balance your biceps and brachoradialis, and make them suffer on the squash court as a result. If you have yourself suffered on the squash court and have a wrist injury, then these exercises can help strengthen your forearm and aid recovery (but remember only to exercise on the advice of a sports doctor).

In practice every exercise where you use your hands will use your forearms, but they are very rarely isolated. Here are a few exercises that will work only the whippets of your wrist, forearm and fingers.

Wrist curls – palms face up

Ever noticed that your writing hand has more of a muscle in the inside of the forearm than the other one? Those are your flexor muscles, and if you want to give them a bit of a strength boost you should try curls with the palms of your hands facing upwards.

In the same vein as working your forearms, don't forget to stretch and strengthen the muscles of your shins and feet – see IDEA 14, *Playing footsie*.

Try another idea...

You can do this with a very light dumbbell, or a tin of beans, or by using a resistance band (see IDEA 31, *Your flexible friend I*). In each case you need to have your forearm resting on a surface, like a table top or a chair arm, with the wrist just over the end and the palm facing upwards. If you have a resistance band you can pin down one end under your foot, and hold the other in your hand. Allow your hand to drop down as low as your wrist will let it and then breathe out and slowly curl your wrist up in an arc as high as it will go. Repeat five to ten times. Now work the other wrist.

Wrist curls – palms face down

These work the extensor muscles along the outside of your forearms. The technique is exactly the same except that you start with the palms facing downwards.

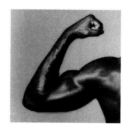

'Forewarned, forearmed; to be prepared is half the victory.'
MIGUEL DE CERVANTES

Defining idea...

205

Twisting

This is hard to do with a resistance band but easy with weights. Simply start with the weight in one hand with your elbow resting on a chair arm or table top and the palm up. Breathe out and turn the wrist over so the palm is down. Reverse and repeat ten times.

Finger flex

We rarely need enormous strength in our fingers but if you do a lot of keyboard work this is a great way to stretch and exercise them. Simply bring your fingertips together and slip a normal rubber band over fingers down to the first knuckle. Now open the fingers up like a flower blooming. Open and close 10–15 times for each hand.

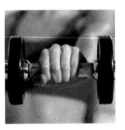

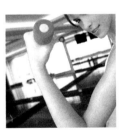

Q **I've found it quite effective to use a small dumbbell for wrist curls with the palm upwards. When I lower the wrist I let the bar roll down my fingers and then roll it back up them again before raising my wrist. I'm told this will strengthen my hand. Is that right?**

How did it go?

A *It is, but remember that the muscles of your fingers are not as strong as the muscles of your forearm and will tire faster, and so you may be tempted to do too many repetitions for your fingers because your forearms don't feel anything. You could always separate the two movements and perform the finger rolling separately.*

Q **I find that my right forearm is fine but my left gets really tired after four or five exercises.**

A *Whichever hand you write with will have much more endurance so for once don't try to make each side do the same exercise. You can try for a better balance between the wrists by working them both, but there will always be a certain inequality unless you are truly ambidextrous.*

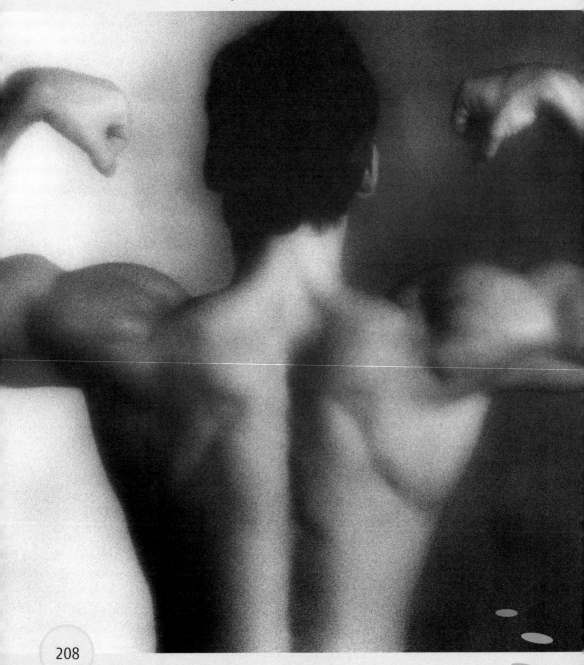

49

Backtastic I

If your back is strong and you don't care who knows it, then here are some more advanced moves to work the back and shape the shoulders.

It's not an easy existence and a strong back and broad shoulders are essentials if you want to make light of life's load. The following exercises are some of the most bionic backbuilders you can hope to do without the benefit of machines.

They are aimed at those who are already confident that they can do the less demanding Pilates back moves and who are looking to connect more deeply with their backs and shoulders while building serious strength into them. Do remember, though, that there's no point getting macho with your moves. It would be pretty poor Pilates practice to spend 99 per cent of the time emphasising the importance of core strength and spinal alignment only to leave you bent over double. Desist at the first sign of discomfort – before you learn the true meaning of 'backlash'.

Here's an idea for you...

Having warmed up with the front and back leg pulls, it's time to go to work with a vengeance by combining the back leg pull and the dip.

Start as normal and pay particular attention to your pelvis. You don't want the little scamp to go AWOL now and have your bum make a break for the mat. Breathe in as you raise your right leg, out as you lower it. Swap legs and breathe in as you raise the left leg, out as you lower it. So far, so good. Now comes the interesting bit. Keeping your body absolutely straight and your pelvis in line, bend your elbows and lower your shoulders towards the floor like a beetle stuck on its back but making the most of it by trying to do a press-up. Unless your anatomy is very unusual it's not your shoulders that will reach the mat first but your buttocks. Straighten your arms to come back up to the start position and go back into the leg-raise routine. It may not sound much but try it and see how comfortable you are with three repetitions of the whole move. Should you have arms and shoulders of steel and wish to make the move harder you can perform the whole sequence with your legs up on a chair.

FRONT LEG PULL

This is both a workout and a warm-up for the following two exercises. Between them they strengthen the lower and upper back, shoulders and the hips.
Start out lying face down on the floor as if about to perform a press-up. Hands should be shoulder-width apart, stomach scooped and pelvis parked in neutral. Go up into the position you would find yourself in at the top of a press-up movement, with your weight now balanced on the toes and the hands. Try not to lock out the elbows. Now breathe in for a count of five as you raise your right leg up off the floor and as high in the air as possible. Breathe out as you slowly lower the leg back down. Breathe in as you now raise your other leg as high off the floor as possible, and breathe out again as you lower it back down. Only your legs should move. Three repetitions of each leg and then move into the back leg pull.

BACK LEG PULL

This is the above exercise flipped over onto your back. Start facing upwards with your arms straightened, holding you off the floor. Your weight should be shared between your hands, which point backwards and away from you, and your heels, which rest on the mat. Take a moment to think about your alignment as the temptation, after years of sitting down, is to allow the bum to sink down. Don't let it, instead make sure your pelvis is in neutral and your whole body in line from the top of your head to your toes. Make sure your abdominals are engaged with shoulders scooped. Now breathe in and point the toes of your right foot while lifting the leg off the mat and as high in the air as you can. Breathe out and slowly lower it back to the start point. Breathe in again as you switch legs and raise your left leg as far off the mat and as high as you can. Breathe out once more as you return to the start position.

Easy peasy? Back and shoulders so bionic they literally shrug off this kind of stuff? Good going. Now look at IDEA 51, *Topsy turvy I*, to take it up a notch and try some even more advanced moves for your back.

Try another idea...

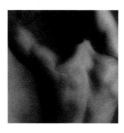

'Pull the other one, it's got bells on'
Traditional take on the gentle art of leg pulls

Defining idea...

How did it go?

Q **I'm trying the back leg pull with dip and it doesn't seem so hard but then I only travel down a few centimetres before I reach the ground. Is that right?**

A   *While it's possible that you have generous curves, which means you bottom out earlier than most, it's most likely that you're starting with your bum out of line. Go back to the position and make sure that your pelvis is lifted high so that it's in line with the rest of your body. That way you should have plenty of travel before your tailbone touches the mat.*

Q **Why do my wrists hurt when I assume the 'back' positions?**

A   *Try changing position. You may be more comfortable if your hands point down the line of your body instead of away from your shoulders. If they still hurt, however, then don't insist. Think about strengthening and stretching your wrists instead (see IDEA 48, Forearm smash) until the exercise feels comfy.*

50

Backtastic II

More workouts for a bionic back and shoulders of steel.

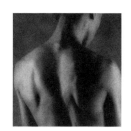

For every Pilates practitioner who's does it because they have had back troubles, there's another who is rejoicing in the strength of their back.

Usually the progression is from back ache to bionic back man, but the reverse is possible: don't try these exercises unless you are totally confident and comfortable with other back exercises.

Following on from the leg pulls and dips of IDEA 49, *Backtastic I*, these are exercises that emphasise the core strength of the back and abs as well as the shoulders. They also form a logical bridge towards the idea of inversion work explored more thoroughly in IDEAS 51 and 52, *Topsy turvy I* and *II*. Here you'll learn to shoulder the weight of the world (well, of your world anyway) and then later you can learn how to turn the whole world upside down.

ROLL OVER

To prepare for this, try loosening up your spine by rolling like a ball (see IDEA 25, *Foetal attraction*). Then lie flat on your back, hands by your side, palms down. Scoop

Here's an
idea for
you... Once you're happy you have the spinal mobility needed to get into position and the
bridge has given you a feel for holding your weight on the feet and shoulders, then it's
time to get to work with the shoulder bridge.

Lie on your back, arms by your sides, knees bent and feet placed firmly on the floor.
Scoop your stomach, park your pelvis and breathe out as you curl your pelvis up from
the floor to lift your whole stomach and hips off the ground. As you do so, move your
hands underneath you and place the palms on your sides or back for support. Your
weight should now be distributed between the soles of your feet and a rough triangle
made of your shoulders, upper arms and elbows, which are all on the floor. Make sure
none of your weight is being supported by your neck or head, the back of which stays
stuck to the floor. Inhale for a count of five as you then straighten the right leg and
raise it so that it is straight up in the air. Exhale as you slowly lower the straight leg
back down to horizontal. Bend the knee and return the leg so the foot is back on the
floor and then perform the same movements but with the other leg this time.
Complete three repetitions of each side.

the stomach, park the pelvis and breathe out as your lift your straight legs off the
floor and try to press your thighs into your chest. Keep the movement coming so
that you roll smoothly and your feet pass right through the vertical and start to
come down over the top of your head until your toes touch the floor (if you can get
that far). You should feel the stretch in your spine, and the further back you can
reach with your feet the more your hamstring will stretch. Remember that this is
about control, not about flinging those limbs out over your head in the vague hope
that they'll wind up in the right position. The slower you can perform this
movement, the better, and the more work it will demand of your abdominals and
back muscles as they strive to stabilise you with your legs in the air.

BRIDGE

Very simply, lie flat on your back, stomach scooped, pelvis parked, knees bent and then, breathing in, lift your pelvis off the floor and raise your back off the ground, vertebra by vertebra, until your body forms a straight line from the knees, down the front of the thighs, the stomach, and chest. Your weight should be shared between the feet and the shoulders. Hold the position for ten deep breaths and then relax to come back down to the ground.

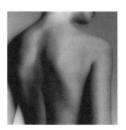

Once you've got the hang of curling your back and taking the weight onto the triangle of upper arms and shoulders, then you can move on to inversion work like the shoulder stand and more challenging back and abs moves in that position. For more details, turn to IDEAS 51 and 52 *Topsy turvy I and II.*

Try another idea...

'It was on my fifth birthday that Papa put his hand on my shoulder and said, "Remember, my son, if you ever need a helping hand, you'll find one at the end of your arm."'
SAM LEVENSON, US humorist, spelling out the joys of self-help when it comes to shouldering problems

Defining idea...

How did
it go?

Q **I get stuck in the roll over and end up staring at my thighs with my legs horizontal. Why?**

A *It could be that you don't have sufficient back mobility: make sure you can perform the rolls in IDEA 25, Foetal attraction, first. If that's not the problem, then it could be that like many of us you don't feel comfortable enough to provide the final push of the hips that sends the legs further out and down towards the floor. It can feel very unstable if you're not used to that triangle of support across the shoulders and upper arms. Check your shoulder and arm position, shut your eyes, and give it a go. You'll be pleasantly surprised.*

Q **Help. I can't get my toes anywhere near the floor in the roll over but I'm sure my back is extremely flexible, so what's stopping me and how do I get over it?**

A *Could be your hamstrings. Men in particular tend to suffer from tight hamstrings and even with amazing spine mobility you won't manage to touch toes to the floor if your hamstrings are too tight to stretch your legs out. Try hamstring stretches and see if things improve.*

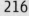

51

Topsy turvy I

Turn your world on its head and reap the benefits for balance and back strength.

Inversion (or standing on your head) is a common technique in various forms of yoga where it is believed to have therapeutic powers for the internal organs, literally taking the pressure off your heart, liver and intestines.

It is also said to have benefits for the blood flow, helping return blood to the heart from the veins. Pilates doesn't specifically refer to inversion, and the more complex yoga headstands don't feature in the Pilates repertoire, but Joseph H. did base a number of exercises around the shoulder bridge – an inverted position directly comparable to the shoulder stands of yoga.

The following are a few moves that will help you get used to flipping your poles.

TOPSY TURVY ZIGZAGS

Before launching into elaborate shoulder stands, try to get a general feel for the upside of being upside down by putting your feet up – right up.

Here's an idea for you...

Happy with the shoulder stand? Then it's time to move on to the full shoulder stand. This is much the same but without the wall and with the legs straight up in the air. It's not easy, and the less practised you are at it the more it'll work your back and abs as you try to balance in position – which is a great workout as long as you already have the strong abs and back needed to do the job. You may want to make sure there's nothing breakable nearby in case our little topsy turvy tower of strength should topple. Start by lying on your back with your legs straight and then place your arms by your side, palms facing down to push against the floor as you bring your bent knees up towards your forehead. As you curl up, shift the weight to the triangle on the ground running from one elbow up the upper arm, across the shoulders and down to the opposite elbow. Use the hands to support the lower back. Keep the back of your head firmly on the floor. When you're stable, with your torso in the air and knees bent, try taking the legs up one at a time by straightening them. Try to stay up long enough to overcome any swaying and stabilise. Believe it or not, you'll eventually find it quite relaxing like this. To get back down, slowly bend your knees back down towards your forehead and then curl your back down one vertebra at a time, shifting your hands from your back to the floor as you come down to provide support and keep control.

If anyone knows of a smooth and suave way of getting into position for this, then please write to me. In the meantime you, like me, will probably have to resort to much bum shuffling before we can get into position close to the wall with our backs on the floor, buttocks at the base of the wall, legs straight and heels touching the masonry. Think about your shoulders and slide the shoulder blades down the spine so your back feels flat on the floor and you can feel the ground between your blades.

Bring your heels together on the wall and now bend your knees a little so you can get the soles of your feet on the wall. Starting feet together, point your toes away from each other to make a narrow V. Then touch your toes to the wall and pivot on them, moving the heels away from each other so your feet point inwards again. Now pivot on your heels and turn your toes outwards again. Reverse the action to bring your feet back to where they where. This increases the circulation, mobilises the ankles and works the small muscles of the shin.

SHOULDER STAND AGAINST THE WALL

This is a halfway house exercise aimed at getting you comfortable enough with shoulder stands to be able to do the full version. Start as above and bend your knees, keeping your feet hip-width apart and the soles flat on the wall for support. Gently roll your spine up from the pelvis and walk the feet up the wall to start lifting your body off the floor and tipping the weight up towards your shoulders. As your bum comes clear of the floor, reach down so that as you lift, your hands are supporting your back and the weight goes onto a V-shape on the floor made from the point of your left elbow, up the upper arm to the shoulder,

Try another idea...

Once you're comfortable with the idea of being upside down, and you've mastered the strength and balance necessary for shoulder stands, then you can move on to try some of the more advanced moves that Joseph H. dreamt up for topsy turvy technique. Take a look at IDEA 52, *Topsy turvy II.*

Defining idea...

'The sound principle of a topsy-turvy lifestyle in the framework of an upside-down world order has stood every test.'
KARL KRAUS, satirist

across the shoulders and out through the other upper arm to the right elbow. Your head rests as it was with the back of the head on the floor, but by the end of the move your chin will be tucked into your chest because your whole torso and upper legs will be vertical with the knees bent at right angles and the feet flat on the wall.

Get a feel for this position and watch for pains in your back or neck. If you suffer pain, then don't persist, just walk away. Of course walking away is easier said than done. To get back to where you were, roll the spine back down onto the floor from the shoulders (remember vertebra by vertebra). Once your bum is safely back on terra firma you can swivel sideways on it and stand up again.

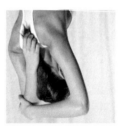

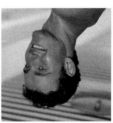

Q   **Should my head hurt?**

A   *No. Although the back of the head rests on the floor it doesn't take any of the weight (that would be dangerous for the neck). Make sure the weight is distributed along that V of elbows, upper arms and shoulders.*

Q   **Feels great. How do I look?**

A   *Good point. Try doing this near a mirror so that (a) you can impress yourself by seeing what you look like and (b) you can spot the fact that your legs probably aren't straight but instead swayed over so your feet are over your face and not in line with your spine. This is a common beginner's problem and you will feel the effort in your abs as you try to correct it and straighten up. Make the effort to straighten and align and enjoy the ab workout on the way.*

How did it go?

221

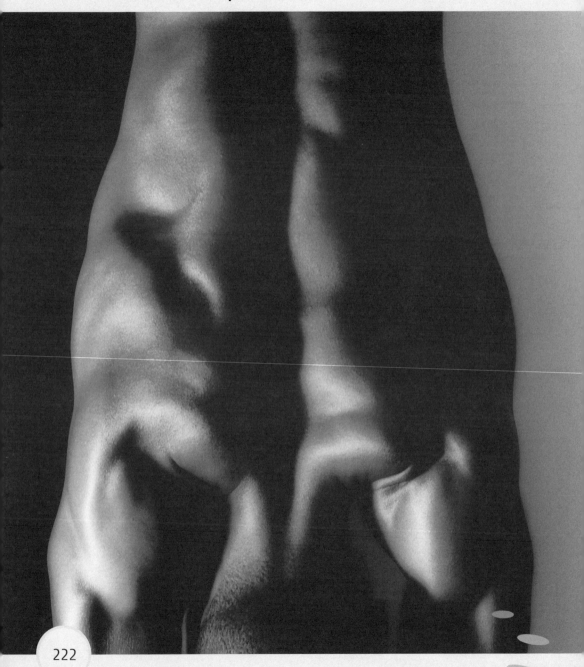

52

Topsy turvy II: Topsytopia

Once you're comfortable upside down, it's time to go to work.

These exercises are all Joseph Pilates' originals. He didn't seem to think it necessary to spend time developing the shoulder stand itself, but us mere mortals will find it really tough just getting into position, let alone working out that way, so make sure you've read Idea 51, 'Topsy turvy I', before you try these.

Many benefits are claimed for inversion work, including improved circulation and the release of pressure on the internal organs. It certainly gives you a different view of life, and the concentration required to get into position and work out is considerable. For that reason I don't recommend that you do the shoulder stand exercises in isolation. Instead, perform them as part of a balanced sequence of stretches and leg/back work. Take a look at the exercises in IDEA 49, *Backtastic I*, for some ideas of suitable preliminaries. Just as important is the mental preparation. Take the trouble to visualise your alignment, to scoop the stomach, watch for neutral (often forgotten when you turn your world upside down), and clear the mind of distractions like work and worries.

Try turning the scissors into the bicycle. Get into the upright position as you do for the scissors and then with your legs in the air start to slowly pedal an imaginary (and upside down) bike. Slowness and smoothness, rather than flailing away, is the key to taking this bike for a spin. Remember that the real work is not being done by the legs (they are primarily stretching the muscles of the groin) but by the abdominals and back.

Defining idea...

'You are old, Father William,'
the young man said,
'And your hair has become
very white;
And yet you incessantly stand
on your head –
Do you think, at your age, it is
right?'
LEWIS CARROLL

JACKKNIFE

This follows on naturally from the roll over in Idea 50, *Backtastic II*, so it makes sense to ensure you are comfortable with that before moving on to the jackknife. It's also a great idea to limber up for this and the following exercises by rolling like a ball (IDEA 25, *Foetal attraction*). Come to think about it, it's a great idea to roll like a ball anyway as it just feels so good.

Lie on your back, hands by your side, palms down, legs straight. Scoop that stomach, slide those shoulder blades down the spine and park the pelvis. Breathe out and sway your legs up to the vertical. Breathe in and check your alignment again, then breathe out as you roll the spine up, one vertebra at a time, starting with the tailbone and tipping the weight back onto the shoulders exactly as if you were performing the roll over but without taking your toes all the way over to the floor. This time it's fine if your legs are parallel to the floor because now you're going to breathe in and snap your legs up to the vertical. From there breathe out as you set the spine back down on the floor one vertebra at a time until you're flat on your back again with your legs in the air. Breathe in and lower the legs to the mat. Perform the whole move three times.

SCISSORS

Start by taking up the full shoulder stand position with your legs straight up in the air and your toes pointed. Place the palms of your hands against the small of your back to provide support; your weight should be distributed across your upper arms and shoulders. Now breathe out as you slowly 'scissor' (split) your legs so that one goes forward and lowers towards your face while the other moves away from your face and towards the floor. Keep the legs straight and the move slow and controlled. Breathe in again and bring the legs back to the vertical, then breathe out and scissor the legs again, but this time the other way so each leg is doing the opposite move to the one it just made. That's one repetition, perform three to five.

For more back and abs work that involves strength and flexibility, take a look at IDEA 44, *Bending over backwards*.

Try another idea...

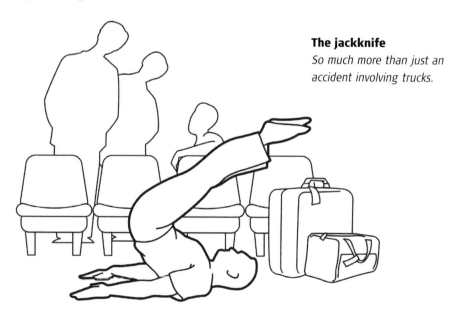

The jackknife
So much more than just an accident involving trucks.

Q **I can't do the jackknife 'snap' without collapsing. What can I do about it?**

A *Simply slow it right down until you and your abdominals are happy about stabilising the movement of your legs from horizontal to vertical. It's a tall order and the faster you do it the harder it is to control, so do it right first and worry about speeding it up later.*

Q **That works a treat – now I have a new problem. I can just about complete the leg 'snap' but I can't hold that position with my legs in the air. What can I do to work on that?**

A *The jackknife is really a combo move taking in the roll over (IDEA 50, Backtastic II) and the shoulder stand (IDEA 51, Topsy turvy I). Try going back to the shoulder stand and just doing that, paying particular attention to the distribution of the weight on shoulders and upper arms. Once you are totally confident of your shoulder stand it's time to go back to the jackknife.*

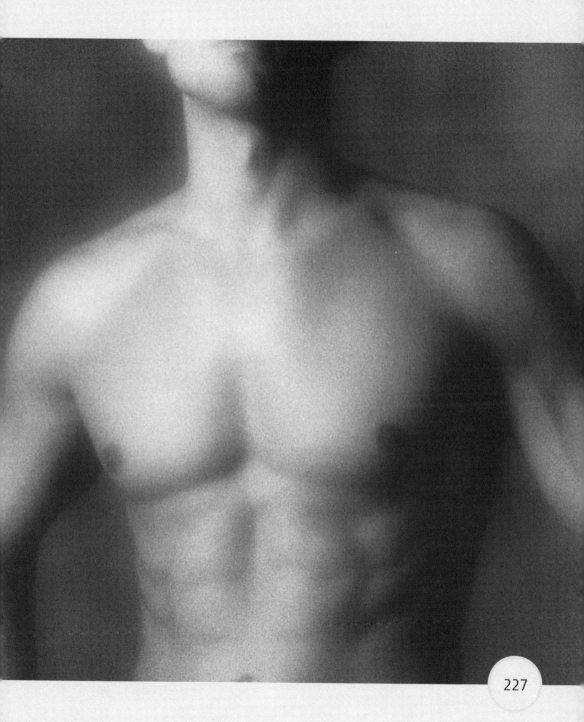

The end...

Or is it a new beginning? We hope that the ideas in this book will have inspired you to try new things and put the spice back into your Pilates. You should be well on your way to a fitter, firmer you, with a fresh spring in your step and a fistful of goals.

You're mean, you're motivated and you don't care who the hell knows it.

So why not let *us* know about it? Tell us how you got on. What did it for you – what helped you punch through the plateaux and beat the boredom? Maybe you've got some tips of your own you want to share (see next page). If you liked this book you may find we have more brilliant ideas for other areas that could help change your life for the better.

You'll find Steve Shipside and the rest of the Infinite Ideas crew waiting for you online at www.infideas.com.

Or if you prefer to write, then send your letters to:
Power-up Pilates
The Infinite Ideas Company Ltd
Belsyre Court, 57 Woodstock Road, Oxford OX2 6JH, United Kingdom

We want to know what you think, because we're all working on making our lives better too. Give us your feedback and you could win a copy of another *52 Brilliant Ideas* book of your choice. Or maybe get a crack at writing your own.

Good luck. Be brilliant.

Offer one

CASH IN YOUR IDEAS

We hope you enjoy this book. We hope it inspires, amuses, educates and entertains you. But we don't assume that you're a novice, or that this is the first book that you've bought on the subject. You've got ideas of your own. Maybe our author has missed an idea that you use successfully. If so, why not send it to info@infideas.com, and if we like it we'll post it on our bulletin board. Better still, if your idea makes it into print we'll send you £50 and you'll be fully credited so that everyone knows you've had another Brilliant Idea.

Offer two

HOW COULD YOU REFUSE?

Amazing discounts on bulk quantities of Infinite Ideas books are available to corporations, professional associations and other organizations.

For details call us on:
+44 (0)1865 292045
fax: +44 (0)1865 292001
or e-mail: info@infideas.com

Where it's at...